HEALED!

A JOURNEY OF FAITH, HOPE, AND MIRACULOUS HEALING

CARL LINDELIEN

DEEDEE LINDELIEN

burning soul press
A STORYSHARING AGENCY

CONTENTS

Cover Design: Dee Dee Book Covers

Paperback: 978-1-964924-07-6
Hardcover: 978-1-964924-08-3
Ebook: 978-1-964924-09-0

"Charm is deceptive, and beauty is fleeting; but a woman who fears the Lord is to be praised." (Proverbs 31:30 NIV)

This book is dedicated to the four most important women in my life. Each day, they bring me joy and happiness!

The first woman in my life is my dear mother, Arleen Lindelien. Not only did she give me birth and a wonderful childhood, but she also encouraged me in everything I attempted to do in my life. Mom believed in me with her whole heart. She also cared for me during the day for the last five years of her life, as only a mother can! Mom read healing scriptures to me from the Bible for hours each day, and she was with me in the hospital daily while DeeDee was at work. I know that she is rejoicing in Heaven today over my healing. You will find her on the corner of Glory Avenue and Hallelujah Street. To God be the glory, forever and ever.

The second woman in my life is my lovely, faithful, dedicated, patient, and wonderful wife, DeeDee. She did not leave me alone during all of my hospital stays. I viewed her in every possible sleeping position and in every type of chair, window sill, or recliner. She never left my side, day and night, in sickness and in health. DeeDee was my voice when I could not speak for myself. She was my advocate supreme! Over the past ten years of caring for me, she has become a registered nurse and doctor for my health care, and she has also been a beautiful wife, mother, and memaw to our children and seven precious grandchildren!

The third woman in my life is my oldest daughter, Shanna Fare, and our three grandchildren, Blake Madison, Noah Wyatt Timothy, and C.J. (Carl James) Nathaniel Bouton. Your love, prayers, and help have brought encouragement and strength to me over the years. Thank you!

The fourth woman in my life is our youngest daughter, Alanna Rae, and her husband, Derek, along with our four grandchildren, Gavin Luke, Grady Lane, Gracyn Rayleen, and Georgia Grace Isaacs. Your love, prayers, hospital visits, and support have been my strength, hope, and joy!

Last but not least, I dedicate this book to God Almighty, Creator of Heaven and the earth, and to my best friend, the Lord Jesus Christ of Nazareth. He suffered and died on the Cross of Calvary to set me free from my sins and the sins of everyone in the world. I thank Jesus because it is by His stripes that I am healed! To God be the glory, forever and ever. Amen!

FOREWORD

BY JIM WIDEMAN

The story you are about to read is true—some of us got to walk it with Carl and his family. The great thing about a book is that now people from all over the globe will get to hear it. May this story minister to you as well.

Jim, is it a victorious story? *Yes!* Is it a tragic story? *At times.* It sure wasn't easy; it took longer than any of us wanted it to. Is it a story of faith? Yes, great faith—enduring faith, mustard-seed faith, mountain-moving faith—but it's also a story of a faithful God who hears our prayers and loves and cares for His children.

I first met Carl over forty years ago at a children's ministry conference in Winona Lake, Indiana. We hit it off instantly. It was like finding a brother who I was separated from when we were babies. Our wives are the best of friends, and our kids grew up together. We vacationed together, went to theme parks together, spent holidays together, ministered together, and brainstormed ideas together. We talked on the phone just about every day. He was a friend who became family!

There has been no one on this earth whom I have said

goodbye to more than Carl Lindelien. Carl had a faith that trusted God no matter what. No matter what the numbers said, no matter what the test results said, no matter what the medical books said, Carl trusted Jesus, the great physician, and Him alone.

I remember him telling me about a doctor's visit he had at the Mayo Clinic. The doctor looked at him and said, "I don't understand it. Most of the patients I see are too weak to shower. They are in a wheelchair and wearing sweatpants. You are shaved and showered, dressed in a suit, drove yourself to this appointment from Minneapolis, and you're going to work every day." Carl trusted Jesus! He was one of a kind!

I never saw Carl discouraged. I saw him tired—I saw him weak and very, very sick—but he always looked at every delay, every setback, as an opportunity to be a blessing to his doctors, nurses, and even fellow patients with the love and care of Jesus. He'd call me from the hospital and say, "Someone in the hospital must have needed me to minister to them."

I learned a lot watching Carl over his twenty-year fight of faith as an adult. One thing he taught me was that you can't control what happens in life. Sometimes bad things happen to some really good people. Yet I watched Carl manage what he could control: his attitude, his words, his joy, his hope, and his faith. He was a wonderful husband and father. His grandchildren adored him. I think everyone who met or knew Carl in any capacity loved him because he loved them first, just like Jesus. He loved everyone.

Carl started writing this book when he first began having serious health complications. He gave me strict orders on what to do to get this story out to others in book form so they could learn what he learned. I pray that it will be a blessing to you. I'm not sure who needs to hear this, but Jesus still heals people today! He's the same yesterday, today, and forever! He hasn't changed!

There's a lot you can learn from DeeDee as well. I remember a minister friend telling me he went to see Carl and DeeDee in the hospital to cheer them up. When he left the visit, he realized that although he had gone to bless them, it was he who was blessed and ministered to by the visit. I told my wife years ago that if anything ever happens to me, be sure and take good wife lessons from DeeDee!

I remember after the Lord healed Carl in 2014, I had the opportunity to travel to Minnesota to minister at some different events. I flew in early so my wife, Julie, and I could go to dinner with Carl and DeeDee. I have to be honest; there were times on this journey when I didn't think I'd have that opportunity. When Carl came walking into the restaurant, wearing a suit and looking his best, it was hard to believe my eyes. The last pictures of him were when he was full of fluid and really didn't look like himself. We laughed, cried, rejoiced, and gave glory to God for what He had done. That's what you did when you spent time with Carl—you left more blessed than when you came, and you left a little closer to Jesus.

In this story, you'll learn about Carl's early life and his family. You'll learn about his first major diagnosis at age fifteen, and you'll see all he went through and what he and DeeDee learned through this fifty-year health journey. Carl lived for almost a decade after the Lord healed him. During this time, he took what the devil meant for harm, allowing the Lord to turn it to good by starting a ministry for those in the hospital and ministering to the hospital staff and employees. DeeDee still leads this today, and she is also a patient advocate.

During the last nine years of his life, Carl told this story over and over in churches, as well as anywhere the Lord opened the door. After he was healed, Carl's heart stopped beating three different times, but he never stopped trusting Jesus. One time, he and I were talking on the phone, and I heard his wife say, "I think his heart stopped." She hung up and called 911. I began to pray for his family and thank Jesus for my dear friend. In about twenty minutes, I received a call from his phone. I thought it was just DeeDee calling us back. It wasn't DeeDee; it was Carl. After the paramedics pronounced him dead and got him in the ambulance, his defibrillator went off and shocked his heart back into rhythm. Carl got a big laugh out of it—he made life better for everyone!

Carl lived to be sixty-five years old, and he enjoyed every minute (and made sure those around him did, too). I sure loved my little buddy, and I miss him terribly!

Maybe you've been on a health journey yourself. Don't give up. What Jesus did for Carl, He can do for you. Maybe you are a family member walking someone else's journey. Take a lesson from DeeDee: God is your source! He's an ever-present help in times of trouble.

In the back of this book is a wonderful list of healing scriptures. Did you know the Bible has a lot to say about healing? Take your time reading each one. Find the ones that jump out at you and speak these out loud over and over—let these promises sink into your heart, not just your head. Years ago, I heard someone quote the Apostle Paul about the good fight of faith. If there's a good fight of faith, there is also a bad fight, so don't fight the bad fight of faith. You are about to experience firsthand what a good fight of faith looks like.

Proverbs 3:5-6 is one of my favorite scriptures. It reminds me of my little buddy's life. It says, "Trust in the Lord with all your heart and lean not on your own understanding; in all your ways acknowledge Him, and He will make your paths straight."

AUTHOR'S NOTES

"YOUR WORD IS A LAMP FOR MY FEET, A LIGHT ON MY PATH." (PSALM 119:105 NIV)

I would like to personally thank you for taking an interest in this book. You probably purchased it because either yourself, a friend, or a loved one is very sick or terminally ill and in need of God's healing power in their body.

Please let me explain something before we get started: this is not a religious book. This book is about a twenty-three-year journey, facing extreme health problems that were much bigger than us.

When each of us is forced to face something, whether it is a giant or an extremely difficult obstacle in our lives, we need help from a higher power, or Creator, who formed us in His own image (Genesis 2:7).

Let me describe to you the health problems that we faced over my entire health journey:

1. Type 1, or diabetes mellitus, for more than forty-one years
2. Legally blind in both eyes (two vitrectomies)
3. Hypoglycemia unawareness
4. Two pancreas transplants

5. One allogeneic eyelet cell transplant
6. Colon cancer
7. Coronary artery disease
8. Two heart attacks and three angioplasty surgeries
9. Acute non-traumatic kidney injury
10. Acute pancreatitis
11. Hyperkalemia
12. Cataracts
13. White blood cell disorder
14. Elevated liver function tests
15. Proliferative retinopathy
16. Peripheral neuropathy
17. Bilirubin excretion disorder
18. Chronic abdominal pain
19. Iron deficiency (anemia)
20. Chronic kidney disease
21. Esophagus varices
22. Aphthous mouth ulcers
23. Gastroparesis
24. Hypertension

As you can see, though some are much bigger than others, my wonderful wife and I faced these health problems together, along with many friends and loved ones who prayed with us and for us, rejoicing in each and every victory over these health issues. Prayer works!

Let me explain where I got my strength and encouragement during this difficult time: the Bible, God's Holy Word! When we face a problem that we need help with, I want to open up a book like no other book has ever been written.

The Bible is always on the New York Times Best Sellers list. Year after year, more Bibles are sold in the month of December than any other book written. The Bible has stood the test of time since the 1600's, with the King James Version of the Bible.

The Bible is infallible; it has no errors, and the books of the Bible do not contradict each other (2 Samuel 22:31, Psalm 12:6, Psalm 119:60, Proverbs 30:5).

The Holy Spirit inspired forty different men to write the sixty-six books—thirty-nine books in the Old Testament and twenty-seven books in the New Testament. These sixty-six books were compiled over a 1,600-year period of time.

Like I said before, this is not a religious book. My prayer is that the scriptures listed in this book bring you hope and encouragement as you put your trust in someone other than yourself (Proverbs 3:5-6).

I would now like to share with you the miracle of healing. I was miraculously healed by God on Father's Day 2014. I did not beg God to heal me. I simply asked Jesus Christ of Nazareth to reach down from Heaven with His healing hand and touch my body. I knew that Jesus had paid the price for my sins and healing on the Cross of Calvary (Isaiah 53:5).

I simply had to release my faith and let my faith join with other believers all over the nation for my physical healing. I know what you are thinking: Did God heal me because of my supernatural faith or the amount of faith I had in his healing power? The answer is no (Romans 3:3)!

Jesus said in the gospels, "Truly I tell you, if you have faith as small as a mustard seed, you can say to this mountain, 'Move from here to there,' and it will move. Nothing will be impossible for you'" (Matthew 17:20 NIV). It is not the amount or measure of faith that heals you. God's will and plan for your life on this earth is what heals you; if you believe in Him.

"And without faith it is impossible to please God."
(Hebrews 11:6 NIV)

I have had many good friends who were believers in Christ, who read their Bibles, released their faith, and were not healed!

I personally believe that each one of us has been given a specific period of time on this earth to do our best to serve Jesus Christ. Some of us have more time than others (Jeremiah 1:5).

I do not know why my friend Perry and his wife Mary lost an eight-month-old baby girl named Melissa to SIDS or why my dear grandmother lived fifteen days short of being one hundred and three years old. What I do know is that each one of us is allotted a certain number of days, months, and years to live a godly life for Christ (Jeremiah 29:11). There is not a specific formula to receive healing. The miracle of healing in our bodies takes place only when it is God's plan for us to be healed. There is no magic formula!

My mother was a believer; she had accepted Christ as her Lord and Savior and was filled with faith. She read healing scriptures to me for six years. My dear mother believed in God for her physical healing, right to the end of her life. My father, my brother Tom, and myself were in the hospice room when she breathed her last breath and was ushered into the gates of Heaven. The New Testament tells us that to be absent from the body is to be present with the Lord (2 Corinthians 5:8).

Pastor Alex and Jeannie Clattenburg at Church In The Son, in Orlando, Florida, were wonderful pastors who were faith-filled and faith-walking. They were former pastors at Calvary in Orlando, one of the largest churches in America. Jeannie wrote and sang over two hundred songs used by churches around the globe, most of them scripture-based.

Approximately a month before Jeannie went to her heavenly home in Heaven, Pastor Benny Hinn from Orlando Christian Center invited Jeannie to come and sing at a citywide crusade he was holding in Arizona. She sang some of the songs that she had written for us. Pastor Benny, along with tens of thousands of people, prayed and released their faith for Jeannie's physical healing from cancer. Was she miraculously healed? No. Was it because of a lack of faith? No. Was it because Jesus stopped healing people? No (Hebrews 13:8).

Our friend Jamie Buckingham was a national leader in the charismatic movement and beyond. He wrote thirty or forty books as a ghostwriter and author, was featured monthly in Charisma Magazine, and had tens of thousands of people praying for his physical healing, yet he was not healed in his physical body.

Pastor Lowell and Connie Lundstrom, evangelists and singers who crisscrossed our nation for more than fifty years, held citywide crusades across America and Canada. They were our pastors at Celebration Church in Lakeville, Minnesota, and DeeDee and I helped them with crusades in their final years of ministry.

Connie beat cancer twice in her lifetime, but the third time she was stricken with cancer, she went to the Mayo Clinic in Rochester, Minnesota, for the best medical care possible. Connie had an ever-increasing amount of faith that grew more each and every day she was alive. She had thousands of prayer warriors lifting her up in their prayers, and she repeatedly spoke healing scriptures over herself. However, this time was different; her work was completed. Connie was not healed in her earthly or natural body—she received her glorified body, like one that Jesus had received after his resurrection from the dead (1 Corinthians 15:42-44).

It is God's will to heal everyone, but I believe that each one of us is appointed a specific number of days. It may be that these days are complete, in which case He simply calls you home for your reward in Heaven.

The other day, I was thinking about the many miraculous miracles of healing in the Bible. Jesus reached out and healed many: the blind, lame, sick, and diseased. Jesus even raised people from the dead: His friend Lazarus, the widow's son, and Jairus's daughter. Everyone that Jesus healed and raised from the dead still died in their earthly bodies!

When Jesus provides physical healing for our bodies, it is not so that we have eternal life on this side of eternity. It is for His glory and honor, so unbelievers can believe!

My journey with Christ for my physical healing in my body has been a roller coaster of a ride, with many ups and downs. My belief in God Almighty, my Creator, and my trust in His Word have not changed. My faith in Christ Jesus as my Lord and Savior has only grown.

I have never been afraid to die, nor have I been desperate enough to try another religion or believe in another god. I simply put my trust in His Word and asked God for help (Proverbs 3:5-6).

When doctors told me the worst news I could hear, I turned to God for help. Sometimes I cried out for help! I released my faith, listened to healing scriptures, and left my physical, emotional, and spiritual healing in God's hands.

My hope is that you will do the same. No matter how desperate you are in life with health problems, please know this:

1. God loves you and knew you before you were formed in the womb. He has a specific plan for you (Jeremiah 1:5).

2. Each of us is given a specific time period to live on this earth.

3. All of us are given a measure of faith to use, putting our trust in God and in His perfect plan for our lives (Jeremiah 29:11).

4. When we pray in faith or cry out to God for help in

desperate measures or extremely difficult times, God hears our prayers (1 John 5:14-15).

5. Sin in our lives can block physical healing for our bodies. Confess any sins in your life (1 John 1:9)!

6. God's will for all of us is to receive physical, emotional, or spiritual healing in our lives (1 Thessalonians 5:16-24).

7. God does not give us eternal life on this side of eternity, but we do receive eternal life in Heaven, where there is no pain, sickness, death, or disease (Hebrews 13:20).

As you read the following chapters in this book, you will see time after time that God heard my cries for help, reached down from Heaven with His healing hand, and touched my physical body.

If you are ill or have a disease like me, and the world's best doctors and specialists in their field have said, "There is nothing more that we can do," you need someone with supernatural powers to help. Cry out to God, confess your sins, and believe in Jesus' sacrifice for your healing on the Cross. Step out in faith, believing in God for your physical, emotional, and spiritual healing.

If this book helps you, please pass it on to others when you are finished reading it. Give it to someone who is in need of God's miracle-working, healing power in their life.

CHAPTER 1
A FIGHTER FROM BIRTH

"I can do all this through him who gives me strength."
(Philippians 4:13 NIV)

It was a cold, windy, and snowy Saturday morning on March 8, 1958. The day brought with it a typical Minnesota spring snowstorm. My mother and father, Ray and Arleen Lindelien, were proud parents of three children: Theodore Merle (Ted), my older brother of seven years, Thomas Raymond (Tom), who was six years older than myself, and Linda, my older sister.

While the wind and snow blew everywhere it wanted and the cold bit any exposed skin, my mother went into labor with their fourth child, which they hoped would be a girl. My parents had wanted to raise two boys and two girls in their young family.

My grandparents on my mother's side of the family, Reverend S. T. and Julianna Thompson, were retired Lutheran ministers. Yes, my mother, Arleen, was a preacher's kid (P.K.). Not a bad P.K., but a very faith-filled woman, who played the organ at church and hosted Ladies Aid (Bible studies), conducted Christmas plays and musicals, held VBS in the summers, and taught Sunday school. My mother gave her all to her church, friends, and family.

My father, Raymond, was also very active in the church. He was the Sunday school superintendent and an usher. Both of my parents loved helping the pastor in the church. My mother had so appreciated the friendships and help that parishioners gave to her parents, especially during the years of the Great Depression.

My parents became best friends with their pastor and his wife at Solar Lutheran Church. Reverend Carl Jensen and his wife tried to have children for years but were unable to become pregnant. My mom and dad told them that if they had a boy, they would give the baby boy to them. This was the "big talk" in the church, and when my dad brought my mother to the hospital in Northfield, they joked about keeping me if I was a girl or giving me away to the pastor and his wife if I was a boy!

My mother went through a fast delivery, and my dad waited patiently in the waiting room at the hospital. Dr. Good, our family doctor, came out of the delivery room and informed him that he was the father of another healthy baby boy! Mother and baby were both doing very well.

Dad, after seeing me and visiting with my mother, decided to go shopping in downtown Northfield for a new electric drill he needed for a project that he was working on. Dad buttoned up his overcoat and lifted up the collar, put on his hat, scarf, and gloves, and drove in the snowstorm a few blocks to the hardware store to make his purchase before the stores closed for the weekend.

It is funny how news traveled so quickly, even in 1958, when almost every telephone call was long-distance and you were billed by the minute. The news was quickly spread to almost everyone in the church on that wintry Saturday afternoon.

On Sunday, when my father and my brothers and sister arrived at church, it was odd because everyone was congratulating the pastor and his wife on their new baby boy!

People in some ways ignored my father, lavishing their attention on Pastor Carl and his wife; the joking around had become real to many people in the church. They had always wanted a boy... However, they did become pregnant after a few months, giving birth to a son and then a daughter a few years later.

My mother and father named me after the pastor, Carl Timothy. They called us boys Ted, Tom, and Tim, as if singing a song! In the seventh grade, I stopped going by Tim, switching to my first name, because I didn't want to be known as Timmy at thirty years old. I am glad that my parents decided not to give me away. My parents did not give up on having another daughter, though, and in two years, Dr. Good delivered my younger sister, Lynette Sandra, into our family.

Our family was growing—three boys and two girls. Life was good, and we were living in a small house on Spring Street in Northfield. Our grandparents also lived in Northfield, on Orchard Street. They lived just across town in a new five-bedroom, two-bathroom rambler.

During the day, my mother worked at Carleton College as a cook, and my dad worked for an Allis-Chalmers farm equipment dealer as a mechanic in the Northfield area. My grandma and grandpa watched my sisters and me while my parents were at work and my brothers were in school.

When I was four years old, our parents bought a five-acre hobby farm south of Lakeville. We enjoyed living out in the country with lots of animals as pets: a horse, goats, sheep, cows, pigs, ducks, chickens, dogs, and lots of cats!

We attended Highview Christiania Lutheran Church, where my mother was the church organist, my dad was over at the Sunday school, and my older brothers were the church janitors. I spent more time at church than the pastor because I followed everyone to church and helped with everything I could.

One of the annual events at Highview was the Christmas program. After all of the Sunday school kids completed the Christmas play, we were given a fresh apple, a bag of peanuts, and some hard Christmas candy, all packaged in a brown paper sack. This was one of the highlights of the year, and that bright red apple was delicious.

My older brothers, Ted and Tom, were in charge of mowing the church cemetery and the lawn. I always followed behind them, appreciative that they would always take me to help them. My job at the cemetery was to trim all of the grass around the headstones. We did not have motorized trimmers back then. What I had to use was a pair of scissors that turned ninety degrees to hand-clip each headstone.

I kept the church alive for years. Each time I would trim the grass at a headstone, I would say a prayer: "Please God, do not let another one die." This prayer was repeated each time I squeezed the handle to trim the grass. There were hundreds of headstones in the cemetery.

Each spring, Ted, Tom, and I went on a week-long fishing trip to the Boundary Waters Canoe Area (BWCA). This is a beautiful series of lakes that extend from Ely, Minnesota, into Canada. If you have never been there, you must make an effort to go. It is gorgeous!

My brothers and I would drive up to Ely, a six- or seven-hour trip, in a blue 1967 Mustang with a long red fiberglass canoe strapped to the roof. Inside the car, we had three back-packs, each loaded and packed with our clothes for the week, camping supplies, some Kool-Aid and pancake mix, a cast-iron pan, and eating utensils. We always ate what we caught, meaning fish, but in the five or six trips we made, I do not think we ever caught one.

I called our BWCA weeklong fishing trip the "Three P's": we paddled from lake to lake, we portaged the canoe and gear to get into other lakes, and we ate pancakes.

In the BWCA, we could drink the water right out of the lake. We camped on the rocky islands rather than the mainland to avoid animals such as bears. And if we kept our eyes open, we would see a small wooden sign nailed to a tree or a signpost saying "Portage" with many rods. This portage was a small trail through the mainland to put the canoe into another lake. The heavy fiberglass canoe we used took at least two people to carry over our shoulders with our backpacks. The lighter aluminum canoes could be carried on the shoulders of one person.

On one of our trips, it rained for four or five days. Our tent was leaking water, our sleeping bags and clothes were wet, the firewood was completely damp, and we had not eaten anything. Tom and I canoed from the island to the mainland in search of dry firewood and anything to eat. We found some dry firewood and loaded it in the canoe. I then stumbled across some wild blueberries and began to pick them furiously. What a find!

With a hat full of blueberries and dry firewood, we paddled the canoe back to the island that we called home, quickly starting a fire. I mixed up the pancake mix with the fresh wild blueberries, and soon we were eating the most delicious pancakes ever. When I think about them, I can still taste them!

After we finished eating for the first time in days, Ted went out in the canoe by himself; the sun had finally started to show itself, and it felt good standing by the warm campfire.

I was looking at the fire when I heard my brother Ted yelling for help. I ran to the edge of the rocky cliff on the island and saw him hanging onto an upside-down canoe. The water was very frigid, and Ted did not have on his life jacket. He struggled in the water, and the canoe drifted further from the island. I immediately jumped off the cliff and into the frigid water. I swam as quickly as I could to the canoe, helping Ted swim it back to the island. Ted said that I saved his life that day. I do not know if I did or not, but I was glad to help him as much as he has helped me. This is what brothers do for each other.

Brothers seem to share something very special with each other. No one else will ever know what it is like to have a brother, except a brother. God made brothers special, and both of mine hold a very dear and special place in my heart.

Both Ted and Tom would take me with them on their dates. Most of them included a movie or two or a "Dusk-till-Dawn" marathon of movies at the Lucky Twin Drive-In. This was a great drive-in movie theater, with two screens that faced each other and the concession stand and projection booth in the middle of the property. After my brothers paid and we drove into the drive-in, my brother and his date would get into the back seat, and I would sit in the front driver's seat to watch the movie. Please note that I did not look in the rearview mirror to see what action was happening in the back seat when the movie got boring! It was great having older brothers; they brought me everywhere, and I was always welcome. Anywhere they went, I was sure to follow.

When I was twelve years old, my parents adopted a child, a girl. My parents turned to Lutheran Social Services, which matched Korean children to families here in the States. It was a matter of months when we received the photo of our new sister, who was ten years old. They named her Elizabeth Suzanne (Liz), and she was the same age as my sister Lynette. My mother could now sing out the girls names, like she had sung out the boys names, when she called us, "Ted, Tom, Timmmm... Linda, Lynette, Lizzzz."

In a few months, we went to the airport to greet Liz. She was flying from Seoul, Korea, to Minneapolis-Saint Paul. We recognized her as she stepped off the plane from the photo we were given. Through an interpreter, the introductions were made, and she was told that we were her new family in America. She knew only one word: "Hello."

The ride home in the car was kind of quiet; we were excited about our new adopted sister but a little scared. This was all new to us. When an infant is born into the family, you get used to them, but Liz was a ten-year-old girl who lived in an orphanage, and we had no idea what her family life (or lack thereof) was like.

I wish you could have seen Liz's eyes when we pulled into the driveway. My brother Tom was raising Springer Spaniels and training them to be hunting dogs. They were housed in the brooder house, with a fence around it. Liz thought we were raising them to eat (I guess they eat dogs in Korea). She wanted nothing to do with us; she loved dogs—not to eat but to have as pets.

Liz was very surprised when she walked into her new home. Mother had prepared some fresh cookies, and we had ice cream with toppings ready to serve. What kid does not like ice cream? Liz did not; she had never tasted it! Everything was brand new for her. My sisters brought Liz the bedroom that she would share with them. She was shown her dresser with her nightclothes, play clothes, and school clothes. I think Liz cried herself to sleep that first night.

When Liz started school with us, she began in kindergarten. Before the end of the year, she was at grade level with Lynette. Liz is a very special person, and she is very intelligent. She became familiar with all of the American trends and fades, adjusting to our culture easily. On the other hand, we did not enjoy her kimchi, a Korean dish produced by digging a hole in the ground, placing vegetables into a container, and burying them for three or four days. After that, it is dug up and eaten with seaweed. I tried it and did not like it, and I usually like everything new, strange, or different when it involves food items.

Liz became a great addition to our family. I love Liz very much, and I am glad to tell you!

When I turned fourteen years old and finished my confirmation class in the spring of that year, I did like most Lutheran teenagers do—I disappeared. After confirmation, you only attend church on a Sunday if you are really sick, get married, or have children and need to bring them to Sunday school. When I was a kid, the Lutheran church did not have much for teenagers.

I do appreciate, however, what the farm men and women taught me: books of the Bible, the Lord's Prayer, the Apostles Creed, the Ten Commandments, the Beatitudes, Psalm 23, John 3:16, the Roman Road, and Bible stories.

All of the years of attending Sunday school, VBS, Christmas plays, and musicals—all of this knowledge and memorization of the Bible—would later help me in the ministry.

I remember the prayers we used to say as a family before meals: "Come, Lord Jesus, be our Guest, and let this food to us be blessed. Amen." As kids, we used to say, "Come, Lord Jesus, be our Guest, and bless this food to Wesley Best. Amen." Wesley Best, our school bus driver, and his wife Beverly lived about a mile from our home, next to the Twin Church Ballpark.

At night, our prayer would be, "Now I lay me down to sleep; I pray the Lord my Soul to keep, if I should die before I 'wake, I pray the Lord my Soul to take. Amen."

CHAPTER 2
INVINCIBILE

"The LORD himself goes before you and will be with you; he will never leave you nor forsake you. Do not be afraid; do not be discouraged."
(Deuteronomy 31:8 NIV)

After Labor Day in the fall of 1972, I began the ninth grade. This was a fun year for me in school. Coach Gene Pressure recruited me to join the swimming team, specifically the springboard diving team. I gladly accepted.

Practicing for the diving team was an exciting and thrilling event in my life. Coach Pressure would pick me up at my home at six o'clock in the morning. We would drive to school together in his 1970 VW Bug, practice for an hour before school and for an hour and a half after school, then he would drive me home. Needless to say, I was in good shape, climbing in and out of the pool after each dive and performing the tricks and twists that each dive required me to perform.

I will never forget the first swim meet that we had at the

new swimming pool attached to the junior and senior high school buildings. The diving competition took place about midway through the swim meet, immediately following the fifty-yard freestyle race. Most of the teams used this as their halftime and would go as a team into the locker rooms, discussing their strategy for the last half of the meet, while the diver's competed in their individual events.

My mother would try to attend every swim meet I dove in. I can still remember exactly where she sat in the spectator stands. I saw her watching me as I climbed onto the board, walked out to the end, and jumped off into the swimming pool. When I swam out of the water for each of the six dives in a competition, I would see her clapping for me.

In March of the new year, my older sister Linda and I flew to Orlando, Florida, to visit Disney World. We flew into the old McCoy (MCO) Airport, just outside of Orlando, and I was shocked. The old airport only had two or three gates, and they would roll the stairs up to the plane so we could disembark. We had to walk outside from the tarmac to inside the terminal to claim our luggage.

This was foreign to Linda and me. We were used to the Minneapolis-St. Paul Airport, which had bridges from the terminal gates right to the doors of the aircraft.

Disney World had recently opened its doors in the suburb of Kissimmee. Orlando was becoming a major tourist destination and would later build a fabulous new terminal at MCO with more than one hundred gates to handle all of the daily flights.

Linda and I stayed at the Hilton Gateway Inn on this trip. One of the benefits of our flying privileges, given to us by Northwest Orient Airlines, was a fifty percent discount at their hotels, which housed the airline employees on layovers. We took full advantage of this benefit and others as we traveled.

The next day, March 8, we went to the Magic Kingdom at Disney World. The parking lot for the Magic Kingdom was larger than all of Disneyland in California. It was an exciting day filled with fun and excitement!

That evening, a little after midnight, Linda woke me up. We stayed at the park until after ten that evening, and by the time we had gotten back to our room at the hotel, it was after eleven. We were tired from a fun and exciting day, and I fell fast asleep as soon as my head hit the pillow. That is, until Linda said to me, "Happy birthday, yesterday!" I had forgotten my fifteenth birthday! What kind of kid forgets their own birthday?

After arriving home from our trip, I took my farmer's license driving test. This was a special license in Minnesota that granted me permission to drive anything, as long as it was during daylight hours. The only time that I could not drive legally was from sunset to sunrise. I passed the driving test with a perfect score, which was easy for me; I had been driving vehicles since I was nine years old.

With this new driver's license, I was able to get long-term jobs and drive myself to school. Paired with a 1964 black two-door Ford Falcon, I landed a job as a dishwasher at a "members only" supper club called The Chart House.

That was one miserable job. The restaurant served a lot of lobster, which meant they had a lot of small, shot glass-type glassware that held melted butter for the lobster. By the time we would get these little glasses to wash with the dishes, the butter was not melted but hard enough that they were difficult to wash. Add to that, the chefs brought their dirty pots and pans to me to scrub. I would be drenched with sweat from the scrubbing of pots and pans, the heat of the dishwasher, and all of the preparation for cleaning the silverware, glassware, and dishware.

I learned a lot at the Chart House and asked a lot of questions to the chefs about the meals they prepared for guests. I did not want to be a dishwasher my whole life! I still remember how I used to scrape out those small glasses of hard butter with my index finger; the smell of the butter makes me sick to this day.

The Village Pantry was a brand new family restaurant that served breakfast, lunch, and dinner. Jerry knew me from Highview Lutheran Church and hired me, not as a dishwasher but as a cook. He had a lot of faith in me, even though I was only fifteen years old. I guess I took after my mother in more ways than cooking.

I learned very quickly how to handle the grill, deep fryers, broasters, freezer, and walk-in cooler, along with the order tickets that would accumulate at ten or twelve every five minutes while we were open. I always treated our dishwashers with respect, asking them if they could please bring me clean dishware to serve the food that I had prepared for guests.

The day after Labor Day, in 1973, I started tenth grade at Lakeville High School. The first three weeks of September were not good; I was late for each one of my classes. After each fifty-minute class, I would go to the bathroom to urinate and then go to the drinking fountain in the hallway and drink water until the bell rang for the next class. I knew something was wrong with my body because the same thing happened at the restaurant. When I went to bed, I carried two quarts of cold water upstairs to my bedroom, only to wake up an hour later from my sleep, walk down the stairs, and enter the bathroom to urinate. This would happen nearly every hour.

I had always been a very healthy and strong kid. I had the normal childhood illnesses like measles, chicken pox, and other common viruses, but this time there was something wrong—really wrong—in my body. I couldn't drink enough water to satisfy my excessive thirst.

During this period of time, I grew weaker and weaker from a lack of sleep and fatigue. The school, my parents, and Jerry, my boss, were concerned with my health. I asked my mother to make an appointment for me with our family doctor, Dr. Roy Good.

I remember the drive to Dr. Goods office that late September day. The sun was shining brightly, and I watched the light clouds float in the deep blue sky against the wonderful fall leaf colors. I was looking at a painting that was supernatural to the human eye. As we drove in Linda's 1965 light yellow Ford Mustang, I do not think that either of us said a word during our thirty-minute drive.

When I arrived at the office, the nurse greeted me and explained that the doctor was running late but would be right with me. Linda and I picked up magazines in the lobby and began to read. Soon, the nurse called my name and informed me that the doctor was ready to see me.

The nurse checked my weight and height on the way to the examination room. Upon entering the room, she asked me what my problem was and why I was there to see the doctor. I informed her of my excessive thirst and frequent urinations during the day and night. She took notes and told me the doctor would be right in to examine me.

When Dr. Good opened the door of the examination room, I stood up to greet him. He asked me about my extreme weight loss since he had last seen me a year ago. After his examination, he instructed me to return to his office in two days for a glucose tolerance test. I would have nothing to eat from midnight on that day, coming to his office fasting until after the test was administered.

The doctor informed Linda, since my parents were not with me and I was a minor, that he suspected I was a Type 1 juvenile diabetic. On the drive back home, we were speech-less, listening to the radio in the yellow Mustang. Linda was driving north on I-35; we were almost half way home when Linda began to cry.

I asked her what was wrong, and all she could say was, "I am sorry, Carl. I feel bad for you. You do not deserve this; you are a good kid." I told Linda, "Do not worry about me. I will be fine." I always thought that doctors fixed the body.

As the north and south lanes of the interstate's split, the most beautiful colored leaves of the trees came into view between the lanes of traffic. The beautiful bright red colors of sumac trees, the golden and bright yellow leaves of maple trees, the many shades of brown leaves of oak trees, and the many shades of green from the leaves that had not yet changed colors brilliantly mixed together!

I can still remember that wonderful day, with the sun shining brightly in the beautiful fall-colored leaves against the deep blue sky. It was breathtaking. How could such bad news be possible on such a beautiful day?

After we arrived home, my mother returned from work, and Linda informed her of what the doctor had diagnosed me with. I remember my mother crying and discussing it with my father. They decided that I should stay home from school so they could watch me closely for the next two days.

Two days after my last visit to Dr. Good, I returned to his office at eight o'clock in the morning. I had followed his directions about not eating; I had not been eating anything for the last two to three weeks anyway. My stomach was full of water, and my bladder really had a workout.

The nurse administered the glucose tolerance test. It involved drinking an orange juice-type drink mixed with sugar every hour for three hours. Blood tests were also taken on the hour and given to the lab for the doctor to review.

The nurse called me into Dr. Good's office for the results of my test. He did not have good news; I was informed that I had failed the glucose tolerance test and that I was a juvenile diabetic (Type 1). He asked me to drive over to the District One Hospital in Faribault and check myself in for treatment and training for the disease that had no cure. Before insulin was marketed in the 1920s, people simply died.

It was only a short mile to the hospital from the doctor's office. After I completed registration, I was told to go up to the third floor, where a nurse would check me into a room. I remember pushing the elevator button and watching the shiny doors slide open. I walked into the elevator, pushed the third-floor button, and watched as the doors closed.

Upon my arrival on the third floor, waiting for me at the desk was a nurse. I do not remember her name, but she had a pleasant smile. She escorted me to my room. I was the only teenager admitted to the hospital that week, so I was given a private room, which I enjoyed.

A short time later, a really old nurse came into my room. She had to be, at least, in her forties, but when you are fifteen years old, that is more than double your age, plus a decade. She was a typical nurse and fit the typical nurse profile: slightly overweight, wearing a white dress, white silk stockings, white shoes, and a white hat in her hair. She had a very matter-of-fact attitude.

The nurse sat at the bottom corner of the bed and began to speak. She told me her name and informed me that she would show me how to test my urine for sugar, give myself an insulin injection (which I would take daily for the rest of my life), and how to eat meals with the diabetic meal plan.

She explained to me what diabetes was and how it affects the body—how you control the disease with no cure.

I was not ready for the words she then spoke over me: "In the next twenty years, you will be dead or blind, have at least one limb amputated, and be in need of kidney dialysis or a kidney transplant."

After speaking these negative words over me, she left to

get the necessary supplies so she could train me on the treatment.

Once she left, I said a quick little seven-word prayer: "Please God, I need a little help!" Sometimes in life, you only have time to cry out for help.

This short little prayer was an indication to God that I was facing something in my life that I could not beat by myself. It was bigger than me, and I needed all the help I could get.

I immediately told myself that the negative words the nurse had spoken over me were not going to stick with me. I accepted the disease, asked God for help, and was convinced that I should remain positive, no matter what happened in my life!

At fifteen and a half years old, my life seemed invincible. Everything that I tried, I was successful at. All of the things I attempted, I conquered. Life was fun, and I enjoyed each and every day. I would face this health problem with positivity, doing my best to set an example for others.

I did not ask God, "Why did this happen to me?" I accepted it, determined that I would live with it, doing my best to be different from all the others I knew who lived with the disease.

A few minutes after the nurse left my room, she returned with supplies. She carried an orange, disposable syringes, alcohol pads, and a vial of saline solution. I was very thankful for the new disposable syringes, which were new on the scene. This meant that you no longer had to boil the old glass syringes to sterilize them before use.

After showing me an example injection, I had to demonstrate the skills by giving multiple injections to an orange. It was then time for me to give myself the first injection of insulin into my body.

The nurse showed me the three locations on my body where I should inject the insulin into my body on a daily basis: the back part of the upper arm, the abdomen, and the thigh. I chose the abdomen location to give my first injection. All I had to do was simply lift my shirt, clean the injection site with an alcohol pad, squeeze the skin together, and inject the needle into the skin. I pulled the syringe plunger back slightly, checking for any blood entering the syringe. If no blood was present, I could inject the insulin into the body. I completed the injection; it was not difficult to perform. The nurse was happy with my success and went on to teach me how to urinate on a glucose urine strip.

There were no blood glucose test strips at that time, except for those used in the laboratories of hospitals and clinics. The urine test strips were very difficult to use. After urinating on a strip, you had to match the color change with five different colors printed on the package. The differences between the first and fifth colors were very close to each other. The spilling of glucose or sugar in your urine was generally ten to twelve hours behind what your actual blood glucose was, but it was the best we had to use in 1973.

My hospital stay was very difficult for me as a teenager. The candy stripers were pleasant to visit with and would furnish me with magazines or books. I did have a television in my room, which I had to pay for. It only had four stations, but there really wasn't much to watch, and back then, the stations signed off until the morning after the ten o'clock news.

There was absolutely nothing to do in the hospital except sleep, but I was not sick; I was feeling great! I wish there would have been a pool table or something for me to do besides read.

I did not wear hospital gowns while I was in the hospital. I wore jeans, a western shirt, and my cowboy boots. I was going to die with my boots on. I did not take them off!

I'd go for a walk, look in the gift shop in the lobby, and on a bright, sunny fall day, I tried to walk outside until the security guard stopped me. The nurse warned him that I might try to escape the hospital. This was not the case; I simply wanted to get out of the stale air inside the hospital building and breathe some fresh air.

Three times a day, a meal tray came into my room. The nurse would accompany it, informing me of how much insulin I should inject into my body to cover the meal. The food was not very good. My apologies to the cooks! Do remember that I was a cook at the time, and a good one at that.

At approximately eight o'clock each evening, the nurses put everyone to bed except for me. I would watch the Tonight Show until midnight and then do something fun while the overnight nurses sat at their desk and gossiped.

One evening, I made my way into all of the rooms, stole the bedpans, and hid them in a hallway closet. As some of you know, the late evening hours are when many patients need a bedpan so that they can go to the bathroom. You should have heard the cries for help from the nurses when they could not find any bedpans to use. (Please forgive me, Lord; I was bored and wanted something to do!) All of the nurses talked about the bedpan incident the entire next day. At least it gave them something to talk about!

After a few very long days, I was released from the hospital, and my mother picked me up and drove me home. My mother had visited me after work each day that I was in the hospital. It was so good to be home and sleep in my own bed, in my own bedroom. Like in The Wizard of Oz, "There's no place like home; there's no place like home."

I enjoyed each and every day of life and lived with a disease that has no cure. I did my best at school, work, and play. I kept moving forward, not looking in the rear-view mirror. I went to school, worked full time, and had fun with everything I was involved in. Two years passed very quickly in my life!

As Labor Day 1975 approached, so did our senior year of high school. The Lakeville School District had just finished building a state-of-the-art, brand new high school for us. We would be the first graduating class from this new building.

As my friend Wayne and I drove my red 1967 Ford Mustang up the long, winding street to the new school building, I parked the car in the parking lot and turned the engine off. I looked over to Wayne, who was sitting in the front passenger seat, and told him, "This year is going to go by so fast; it will be as fast as a blink of an eye."

This year, we were on the work experience program. While Wayne did not work very often, slipping from one job to another with many months in between jobs, I, on the other hand, started a janitorial job in the warehouse of Merillat Cabinet Company.

I had a great boss, and he required that I clean his office, the bathrooms, and the lunch room every day. After I finished washing all of the windows, I would simply sweep the warehouse until it was time to leave for the day. It was not a glamorous job, but it paid well, and it was something easy for me to do.

CHAPTER 3
FROM MEETING TO MATRIMONY

"He who finds a wife finds what is good and receives favor from the Lord."
(Proverbs 18:22 NIV)

In February 1976, my mother planned a trip to Orlando, Florida, with my two younger sisters. Mom asked if I would go with her, knowing that she would have a miserable time with my two little sisters (all they were interested in was boys). My mom liked to have fun on her vacations, and so did I. We loved a well-planned, adventure vacation together.

We were great travel companions and enjoyed trips to: Acapulco, Mexico, to watch the cliff divers and dive; Mexico City, to view a bullfight; the Gulf of Tehuantepec, to water ski; and Acapulco Bay, to parasail.

My mother and I loved traveling to Oahu, Hawaii. We visited Pearl Harbor to pay our respects at the USS Arizona Memorial to those who gave their lives on December 7th. We hiked up Diamond Head, rented a VW Thing, and drove around the island, stopping at pineapple fields and enjoying the plants, trees, and spectacular views. We always stayed right on Waikiki Beach. We saw the legendary Hawaiian singer Don Ho in concert, and, of course, we enjoyed the evening luaus.

Mom and I visited Sacramento to visit with relatives, San Francisco to ride the streetcars and visit Alcatraz, and Los Angeles to watch them broadcast television shows like The Price Is Right and The Tonight Show, starring Johnny Carson.

So when she asked me to go with her on this Florida trip, I said, "Absolutely!" It was a wonderful trip; the weather was fantastic (the weather in Minnesota is not very nice in February). We enjoyed Disney World very much, and on our last day, we decided to stay at the Hilton Gateway Inn swimming pool for the day. It was a good thing!

I was showing off my diving skills on the diving board, wearing my red and white striped Speedo diving suit from the swimming team, when I saw a beautiful girl talking with my sister Liz. This girl was absolutely beautiful!

As I walked over to Liz, I asked what the girl wanted. Liz told me she asked her if we were boyfriend and girlfriend (remember, Liz is my adopted sister from Korea). Liz told her no; we were brother and sister. It was time for me to make my move on this wonderful, beautiful girl.

I walked over a few steps and began a conversation with the most beautiful girl I had ever seen. I asked her what her name was. She told me her name was DeeDee. I introduced myself as Carl, sharing that I lived in Minnesota, to which she replied that she was from Queens, New York City. I asked if she would like to have dinner with us that evening in the hotel's restaurant. Thankfully, she said yes!

We had a wonderful time together at dinner and decided to go to her room after to play cards. We visited until the wee hours of the morning, when we decided to go for a walk to the Howard Johnson Hotel for ice cream at about two o'clock in the morning.

After walking back to the Hilton, we visited the swimming pool until the sun rose the next morning. My mother, sisters, and I had an early morning flight out of Orlando. I told DeeDee how glad I was to have met her and wrote down her address and telephone number, telling her that I would visit her one day in New York City. I said goodbye and gave her a quick kiss on the cheek before leaving for the airport. I wrote DeeDee a letter on the airplane. I had never met anyone like her in my life. She was amazing!

When I got home, I mailed the letter, and a week later, I made a long-distance call to New York City. DeeDee was not home at the time, so I left a message with whoever answered the phone at her home. I told her to give me a call when it was convenient, leaving my telephone number with whoever answered the phone.

At this time, I enjoyed playing pool at a bar in Elko. I was eighteen years old, which was also the drinking age, so I was allowed to go into the bars and play pool. When I arrived home that evening after playing, my mother told me that DeeDee had called.

I immediately called DeeDee back, forgetting that they were on eastern time, one hour ahead of us. I think I woke her up, but we talked for a long time, and I planned a trip to New York City in two weeks. It would be one of my three-day weekend trips I would take monthly. I was very excited to plan this trip. I was really looking forward to seeing DeeDee again—I believe that it was love (or lust) at first sight!

DeeDee and her nine brothers and sisters lived in the Queensborough Bridge Projects. This was located underneath the Queensborough Bridge, which was the thoroughfare to the island of Manhattan. Upon my arrival, DeeDee gave me a big hug, and I was quickly introduced to her brothers, sisters, and parents. Her uncle, Nick, had accompanied her on the trip to Florida, so we quickly caught up on all the happenings from the last month.

Uncle Nick was friends with a very sick man named Robert. He wanted to give a boy and a girl from the projects an all-expenses-paid trip to Florida—specifically Disney World and a trip to Puerto Rico—before he died. Uncle Nick told Robert about his nieces and nephews, and it was decided that DeeDee's older sister, Angel, and her brother, Johnny, would go on the trip.

At the last minute, Angel got scared of flying and bowed out of the trip. DeeDee took her place, and I am very glad she did! It is funny how I was not planning on making the trip either, but both of us were last-minute replacements.

I believe now that God had a plan for us to meet, fall in love, get married, and raise a family! Many times, we do not know why or how something is happening in our lives, but it is all in God's infinite plan for our lives.

My three-day weekend in New York City was fun and exciting; I loved spending time with DeeDee and her family. On my return flight, I could not stop thinking about her, even writing another letter telling her how much I enjoyed our visit together. At the close of the letter, I extended an invitation for DeeDee, Uncle Nick, and Robert to visit me in Minnesota in the near future.

It was now in early April of 1976. I was working hard, saving my money, and preparing for high school graduation in the first week of June. Time was really moving fast, and I was enjoying each and every day.

DeeDee and I had a long-distance relationship, which profited Ma Bell because we had to pay long-distance charges by the minute. I wrote DeeDee a letter every other day, and I called her on the telephone so I could hear her wonderful, special voice. I could spend hours on the telephone with DeeDee, just listening to her voice.

I planned another trip to New York City, planning it out to enjoy DeeDee's company.

Upon my arrival at LaGuardia Airport, I hailed a cab, and it dropped me off at Uncle Nick and Robert's apartment. DeeDee was waiting for me there. I was a little apprehensive about approaching her, but she ran to me, giving me a big hug, a short kiss on the lips, and telling me how much she had missed me.

The next three days were amazing, exciting, and filled with fun! We went shopping on Steinway Street, went to a movie, and enjoyed meals at restaurants that DeeDee loved. We walked and talked, spending almost every waking hour together. Many times we would simply listen to records at the apartment, where DeeDee would pretend that she was Diana Ross as she sang with the Supremes' records. She was an excellent dancer and a good singer, and her choreography was outstanding! It was so much fun for me to watch her sing and dance to the music.

DeeDee tried very hard to make me a dancer. She attempted with all of her heart to show me the dance steps for "The Bus Stop," "The Hustle," "Y.M.C.A.," and "Freak Out." I was not very good with dancing to any of these popular songs—it seems as though I have two left feet! I did, however, take a square dance class in junior high school, but DeeDee was not interested in "Swing Your Partner." She was a city girl, not a country girl, and that is one of the reasons why I was so in love with her. I love the way she walked, the way she talked, the beautiful smile on her face, the joyous laughter from her lips, and her beautiful eyes that could look right through you and into your heart.

It was now the third day of my weekend trip. I enjoyed every moment that I had spent with DeeDee and did not want to leave her alone again. A small, still voice inside told me to ask DeeDee a question. I opened my mouth and spoke these words to DeeDee: "Would you like to travel with me tonight back to Minnesota and live with me? I mean, would you like to marry me?"

DeeDee looked into my eyes and responded back, "Yes! Yes, I will!"

With this response, I had to go to DeeDee's mother and father to ask them for her hand in marriage. However, our meeting did not go well. Anna, DeeDee's mother, wanted all of her children to live within a mile or two of her for the rest of their lives. When she was informed that we were leaving New York City to live in Minnesota, she wanted nothing to do with me! The old Italian families lived very close to each other so the mother could always have her finger on the family.

I called my mother on the telephone, asking her what I should do. My mom was great at solving problems. She asked me if I had enough cash with me to buy DeeDee a one-way ticket. I did, so she told me to take the last flight out of New York that evening with DeeDee and that we would sort things out after our arrival back home in Minnesota.

It was a wild few months. We were two young, dumb kids in love. We moved fast, trying to sort things out. Looking back, maybe we moved too fast, but it all worked out because somewhere amidst the crazy. We gave our lives, plans, hopes, and dreams to our Heavenly Father. We quickly found ourselves dating, engaged, married, and about to become newlywed parents. DeeDee kept in touch with her New York family as well as we could on a limited budget; we called at least once a month and wrote often. No matter how much resistance we felt, we pushed through to keep them in our lives, and it worked. After years of them seeing our love for each other and our love, trust, and faith in Jesus, DeeDee's parents finally came to visit us in Minnesota. It was then that we got to pray with them and introduce them to Jesus Christ.

When DeeDee and I found out we were expecting our first child, we did not know what we were going to have—a boy or a girl. It did not matter to us, as long as the baby was healthy. On August 3, 1977, at 3:33 a.m., we had a beautiful baby girl, weighing in at eight pounds and three ounces (on 8/3/77, that is!). We named our little girl Shanna Fare.

Three years later, our little family grew again as we expected our second child. Once again, we did not want to know if we were going to have a boy or a girl; we only wanted a healthy baby.

It wasn't a boy; it was another beautiful baby girl born on July 19, 1980. We named our second daughter Alanna Rae. She weighed seven pounds and two and a half ounces. DeeDee and I were very proud parents of two very special girls, whom we love with all of our hearts.

We were very busy with work and play, but we always took time from our day to be with our family. I loved coming home from work. When I arrived, Shanna would greet me at the door with an apple to eat, asking me how my day was.

DeeDee and I started attending a church when I had a day off. I would attempt to take Sundays off so I could spend time with my family. They were everything to me. I wanted to be a great husband to my wife and a great father to my children.

Farmington Assembly of God Church met at the local high school on Sunday mornings. The church was pastored by Jerry and Kathy Strandquist, along with the youth pastors, Rod and Melody Carlson. Both of our pastors were outstanding in their jobs. We were the largest Full Gospel church located south of the river.

I always enjoyed Pastor Jerry's sermons. They were based on issues of the current day and how believers should present themselves as Christ's ambassadors to the world. I especially enjoyed the quiet time of the sermon presentation; I used it to gather my thoughts and write down my goals for the week, month, and year. We felt very loved and appreciated at the church.

DeeDee and I would always try to slip out of church during the upbeat song at the end of the service. Pastor Strandquist would meet me near the lockers in the hallway of the school to shake my hand, telling me to have a great week.

After several months of attending church, we got involved in the cooperative nursery and in teaching Sunday school for the toddlers. This was the beginning of us realizing the calling on our lives to be in ministry. All I knew was that Jesus was changing us on the inside to love Him and others more. The more we served, the more we wanted to serve, and the more blessed and fulfilled we became!

Life was good; Jesus was making a difference in us, and we wanted to learn all we could about Him and His plan for our lives. Trusting Him made the difference, but we had no idea of the journey ahead and how it would affect our whole family.

CHAPTER 4
DON'T GIVE UP

"Remain in me, as I also remain in you."
(John 15:4 NIV)

Even when God is good, life can still be hard. DeeDee and I were learning a lot about Jesus and doing life together. Things were good, yet I still had Type 1 diabetes. I learned how to live with the disease and how to treat myself with a proper diet and exercise plan, along with giving myself daily insulin injections.

DeeDee and I were the proud parents of two beautiful little girls. They were our life! Both of us were trying our best, with God's help, to be the best parents possible for our girls. I also wanted to be a better provider for my family—to not have to travel for work and be absent as much as I was at my present job.

I resigned from my maintenance position at ValleyFair Entertainment Center to take a job selling cars at Grossman Chevrolet in Burnsville, Minnesota. The Holy Spirit led me to take the job during the worst year for car manufacturing and sales, but I was obedient in following the steps directed by God Almighty.

While working at the dealership, I made friends with a middle-aged man named Lenny, who also worked as a salesman. Lenny and I did not choose this to be our profession; we were simply doing this job for a period of time to put food on our tables and provide for our families.

Lenny, after four or five months, landed a job with the Rayloc Brakes Corporation. He was a territory manager for Napa's Distribution Center in Minneapolis.

A month or two later, Lenny called to inform me that there was a manufacturer's representative position available with New Britain Tools, and he gave me the number for the person to contact about the job. I called about the job and talked to Ron Rieter, the person who had been the representative for twenty years. He was very interested in me, quickly setting up an interview time to meet. After the interview, he asked if I was a Christian; I told him I certainly was. It turns out that he and his wife were as well!

Ron hired me, and I took over his old territory with a lot of help from him. I was given a brand new car to drive, paid family health insurance, an air travel credit card, and a rental car credit card from the company. Plus, I was given a great salary and bonuses paid for achieving quarterly and yearly sales goals.

With Ron's help and encouragement, I became the salesman of the year for Litton Industries—New Britain Tools. At that time, Litton Industries was the largest conglomerate in the world. They owned everything from Navy shipbuilding companies to noodle factories. You may even remember the Litton microwave ovens from the early 1980s.

I was very thankful for this new opportunity to better myself and provide for my family. I didn't realize at the time that this job change was preparing me for the ministry and working alongside all types of people with different personalities and work ethics. I really enjoyed meeting all the new people I was working with, especially the CEO, John Creighton. John taught me things I didn't know I needed to learn. He was the first leader I had ever worked for who would admit when he made a mistake. I learned a lot from his leadership style and his integrity, but many more changes were ahead for me.

Within a few months, a man in Dallas, Texas, purchased our company, and the cutbacks came at us quickly. There were only twelve of us left in our company after it was purchased, but for some strange reason, I had peace that the Lord was in control. We were asked to meet with the new owner at our distribution center in North Carolina.

During the meeting, he looked each one of us in the eyes as he asked, "Are you with me?" With a holy boldness, I replied, "No," after hearing a small, still voice inside my spirit. "Why?" he asked me. I told him that I believed God was calling me into the ministry, and my yes was to God's plan for my life.

He asked me to stay on board to put out fires with the other brand names wherever needed. I decided that I would do this for him, and he agreed to pay my salary for nine months, let me keep the leased vehicle, still turn in my expenses on a weekly basis, and keep all of my benefits. This was a tremendous blessing for my family.

I was volunteering at our home church with Pastor Jerry and Kathy Strandquist. DeeDee and I were working in the children's ministry and loved every minute of it. For a nine-month period of time, I worked from my home office, volunteered at church, and completed my Bible training through the Assemblies of God. God provided for my family, and we were blessed beyond all measure.

In my management training, I was taught to make your

job indispensable to the company, guaranteeing a position for you. This is what happened with DeeDee and myself at the church. Our ministry and the call of God in our lives put us in a position to be on the ministerial staff. We had a radical life-style change after joining the staff at the church. I was used to a six-figure income with the benefits package; now I made one hundred dollars a week with no benefits.

From that time to now, I never again made the income that I did in the corporate world. Yet, God provided for every one of the needs in our family. He did not always provide our wants, but He supplied all of our needs. Ministry is about saying yes, not about making money. Jesus was teaching me I could trust Him, which was a lesson I would need as I walked out my healing. The more I trusted Him, the more I became sensitive to His leading.

After serving for several years, I sensed a change was coming for me and my family. I accepted a new ministry opportunity to serve in a new church plant in St. Cloud, Minnesota, under Pastor Wes Brooks. I was excited to help him pioneer this new church. It was there that I realized we were also to disciple two young boys—Jamie Doyle and Big Al Florek—in the children's ministry. Both of them went on to pursue ministry as well.

The church continued to grow and God was using us, but, again, I sensed a restlessness that I recognized from before—I knew another assignment was about to open for us.

Soon after this, we moved from St. Cloud, Minnesota, to Biloxi, Mississippi, in obedience to God's calling on our families lives. God truly blessed our ministry at Cedar Lake Assembly with Pastor Kenneth and Joyce Broadus. They were very good ministers, and we became very close with them. Our family would even go on vacation together. *Who goes on vacation with their boss?* We did, and we enjoyed every minute of it! Pastor B. taught me everything he knew about people and ministry; he poured his life into me!

After almost four years of our ministry here, *Charisma Magazine* wrote an article featuring our children's ministry. Unfortunately, after this publication, we experienced "church drama" due to jealousy. I did not want to see this drama cause a church split, so I resigned my position, knowing God would take care of us and honor our commitment to pursuing peace.

Mr. Steven Strang was the CEO, owner, and publisher of Charisma Media in Lake Mary, Florida. When he found out about my resignation, he asked me to come to Florida to interview for the position of New Projects Editor at Charisma Life Learning Resources. They were starting a new Sunday school curriculum for charismatic churches to use.

I ended up serving with them on an advisory council for this new curriculum, working closely with Kim Terrill, who was the sales and marketing manager. Kim and I became very good friends. After a short time, a position opened to lead the creation of this curriculum.

I found myself interviewing again, and I was hired for the position. My family and I headed to the land of Mickey in Orlando, Florida! Steve and Joy Stang were great to work with. I helped with editing and hiring writers for the curriculum, and I created a new kid's church curriculum called K.I.D.S. (Kids in Divine Service) Church. We sold over five thousand units of the curriculum to churches.

While working at Charisma, I had many opportunities to consult and help churches with their children's ministry. Pastor Alex and Jeanie Clattenburg in Orlando asked me to consult with them on a new church they started in downtown Orlando. After consulting with them for several months, we were invited to join the ministerial staff at Church In The Son part-time, in addition to working at Charisma.

I would do anything for Pastor Alex; he had a vision to reach people like no one else I had ever met. I helped him in every way I could to make the vision God had given him a reality for the community of Orlando, Florida.

One bright, sun-shining day, my oldest daughter Shanna was riding home with me from church in my car when I noticed something like a spider web in my right eye. I removed my sunglasses, cleaned the lens with my shirt, and tried them on my face again. I saw the same spider web. I took my glasses off again, asking Shanna if she saw anything in my eye. She could not, and I closed my left eye to concentrate on what was happening in my right eye.

After exiting the interstate, I drove home to tell DeeDee what was happening with my eye. She called the emergency room at Florida Hospital, and they informed me that I should see a retina specialist as soon as possible, which I did the very next day. I called and got an appointment to see a retina specialist in Orlando.

That evening, I prayed to God and asked Him "for a little help with my vision." It was getting cloudy to the point that I could no longer see out of my right eye. I could not sleep the entire night—the enemy was attacking my mind with negative thoughts. I realize now that Jesus was teaching me how to fight the good fight of faith, not relying on what I saw in the natural world to dictate what I believed.

At this point, I had only visited a doctor three or four times in the last twenty years. My life was going great; I was healthy and did not have the problems that I was told I would have at fifteen years old.

My daughters did not even know that I was diabetic. They sometimes noticed that I acted drunk or slurred my words, which is a sign of hypoglycemia, or low blood sugar. I would take a piece of candy from one of the candy dishes placed around our home and office, or they would see me drink some orange juice and be fine. They knew that I did not eat certain foods and that I only drank Diet Coke or black coffee, but they did not know that I gave myself daily insulin injections and tested my urine multiple times a day.

When I arrived at the eye specialist the next day, the doctor examined my eyes and took pictures of them with a computer. This was to show me what was happening with my eyes. Small blood vessels in the cornea had started leaking blood into the clear fluid that holds the cornea in place in your eyes.

He informed me that if I could not see out of the eye, he could not see in the eye to treat the blood vessels with laser surgery. He asked me not to strain myself physically because this would cause more bleeding. In a few days or weeks, the fluid should clear up, and I would be able to see out of the eye again.

This was true, and in a few weeks, I returned to his office and had my first of many laser surgeries performed on my eyes. Over the next five years, I had hundreds of laser surgeries to seal leaky blood vessels in my retinas.

I took everything in stride, kept a positive attitude, and did not tell others about my visual problems. I did, however, remind the Lord that He was my healer (Psalm 107:20).

My eyesight grew worse and worse. It was fine if it was bloody with only one eye at a time, but when both eyes started bleeding at the same time, this limited everything I did and made it more difficult to minister. I was so thankful to God when my eyes would stop bleeding and things would return to normal for a day or two each month. This went on for four years of my life, but this would all soon change as I embarked on the biggest health giant I had ever faced.

One day, I had to return to Tulsa, Oklahoma, to pick up a Harley-Davidson motorcycle I had purchased. I was to fly to pick it up and drive it back to Orlando.

When I boarded the aircraft, I noticed my good eye was starting to leak blood. My other eye was already very cloudy, and I could not see anything but images that looked like shadows. I tried to find my assigned seat on the airplane, but I could not see the seat numbers posted below the overhead bins. I asked the flight attendant for some assistance, and I sat down to pray like I had never prayed before. I prayed the whole way to Tulsa, Oklahoma, without ceasing.

When I arrived at the Tulsa airport, I was very familiar with the layout of the airport complex because I had flown in and out of the airport a lot. My friend was going to pick me up at the airport but had gotten delayed, so he sent his mother to pick me up. She recognized me and said, "Hello Carl, over here!" It was a good thing she said something to me, or I would have walked right by her, not being able to see her standing next to the door.

I followed her very closely to her car and opened the back door, putting my carry-on in the back seat of the car. It was then that I heard a voice standing right next to me, asking, "Would you please drive the car to my home for me? I get nervous driving in all of this traffic in Tulsa." She slipped her key ring into my hand, opened the passenger's front door, and sat down in the seat. What was I going to say to this dear woman?

I told her that I would be happy to drive her car home for her.

I was stepping out in faith, putting my trust in the Lord God Almighty. I exited the parking ramp from the airport many times, so I knew the layout of the parking ramp by heart. This would not be that hard for me! When I closed the driver's side front door, I said a quick prayer, silently asking God for "a little help, please!" I stuck the right key in the ignition and started the engine. I backed out of the parking spot very slowly, trying desperately to look out of my bloody, cloudy retinas.

I looked at the painted plywood signs hanging from the fences in the parking lot, desperately trying to figure out where to go, but I could not read them or tell which direction the arrows pointed. I told my friend's mother that I could not drive her home safely with my current eyesight, so she traded spots with me.

When we arrived at her home, I asked her if I could spend the night, believing that God would heal my eyes while I slept before I needed to ride my motorcycle home to Florida. She was happy to host me, and she quickly showed me where I could sleep that night.

Once again, I did not sleep well that evening. I prayed continually and confessed sins to God—even ones that I had never committed—just to be safe! I was desperate for divine healing in my eyesight from Jesus Christ. I had no one else to trust or turn to in my life.

When I awoke in the morning, I was asked how my eyes were. I stepped out in faith, not by sight, by replying, "Much better!" I hung around the house as late as I could without being a bad houseguest. I drank coffee and visited with my friend until he had to leave for work, which left me alone with his sweet mother.

I put on my leather chaps, jacket, and helmet, started up the motorcycle's engine, and let the engine warm up as I stared into the horizon, trying to view the country roadway in front of their home. I could see images or shadows of green, which were the ditches of the gravel roads, but I could not read the directional or informational signs posted along the roadways. I knew what the shadow of stop signs looked like, so I stepped out in faith, or rode out in faith, down the back roads of Oklahoma into Arkansas, praying all the way.

It was remarkable how God healed my eyes as I continued

riding my motorcycle through the small little towns dotting the back roads. I did not want to travel on the interstate; it was too congested with traffic and people driving way too fast for me and my very limited eyesight. As the day grew longer and the sun shone brightly against my sunglasses, God continued to slowly restore my eyesight while I rode through the back roads of Arkansas into Mississippi.

On Saturday, I visited the Harley-Davidson store owner in Jackson. The owner quickly repaired the alternator on my bike, and I was off to Florida again. The fluid in my eyes began to clear, and I was able to see most of the highway signs. God was restoring my eyesight as I continued to walk in steps of faith.

Many times, in my life and in the lives of others, God heals us slowly as we begin to walk or step out in faith. Some of us, because it is not instantaneous healing, forget to thank Him for His miracle-working power on the Cross of Calvary.

CHAPTER 5
A MOVE BACK TO MINNESOTA

"For we are God's handiwork, created in Christ Jesus to do good works, which God prepared in advance for us to do."
(Ephesians 2:10 NIV)

In February 1998, I received a telephone call at our home in Florida from the evangelist and pastor, Lowell Lundstrom. Pastor Lowell and his wife Connie, along with their oldest daughter Londa, had started a new church plant in Burnsville, Minnesota, called Celebration Church.

Pastor Lundstrom asked me to travel to Minnesota to visit and attend the Sunday services, which were currently held at the Mraz Theater in Burnsville High School. I had no interest in doing this. Our family had lived in the south for the past twelve years. We did not have to shovel snow and withstand the very cold winters of Minnesota. On Thanksgiving and Christmas Day, we would go to the beach or swim in our pool!

I had been with Pastor Alex at Church In The Son in Orlando, Florida. We had to set up for church each Sunday and for mid-week services in rented facilities. Setting up for each service in different locations was very difficult for us. After a little more than three years of this, I did not want to return to this type of church. I wanted to go to a church that had a well-planned-out and functional building.

I told Pastor Lundstrom that I wasn't interested in the position, but a few days later, I received a telephone call from him again. He asked me to check out the church and to advise him on the children's ministry for the church. He had found out that my parents lived only thirty minutes from Burnsville, so he encouraged me to come visit my parents at the same time. This sounded good to me!

I agreed to fly home to Minneapolis, spending four days with the leadership team of the church and also visiting with my parents. It was a great trip, but I didn't want to live in the snow again. After saying no to his offers, we flew back to Florida, and God began to speak to us about how His direction was better than our own wants. After much prayer, I called Pastor Lowell, agreeing to talk about the vision for children's ministries at Celebration Church.

Do you remember how my eyes were still bleeding from my retinas? I had over one hundred laser surgeries on both of my eyes. At times, I was legally blind. I could not view a six-inch "E" held six inches away from my eyes. Sometimes, I had clear vision in at least one eye, but many times, both eyes were cloudy, which impaired my eyesight dramatically. I did not tell anyone about my visual problems, except DeeDee. I continued to step out in faith.

After a year of ministry at the church, my eyesight was so bad that I could not see any facial details on people's faces. I had become very good at recognizing people by their voices.

DeeDee found a retinal specialist in St. Louis Park, about an hour's drive north of the church. I went to visit Dr. Kirk

Morgan at his office, and he examined my eyes. I was surprised by the words from his mouth: "I can fix your eyes, one at a time."

What an answer to our prayers! For years, we had lived with my visual problems. Our prayers were spoken many times, night and day, for the last five years.

Within six months, God and Dr. Morgan restored my sight to 20-30 in both eyes. After the vitrectomies (eye surgeries), cataracts formed, so I had cataract surgeries in both eyes, and new artificial lenses were installed. I am glad that God uses doctors, medical staff, equipment, and medicine to heal our bodies. *Jesus is the great physician!*

With my eyesight restored, I thanked God each time I opened my eyes and was able to see the alarm clock. When we lose something of great value in our lives, it makes us appreciate the little things in life, like our eyesight.

If God had not moved us back to Minnesota, I would still be legally blind. The medical care in the Twin Cities is the best in the world, with the Mayo Clinic in Rochester and the University of Minnesota Hospital in Minneapolis, along with Abbott Northwestern and Regions Hospital in St. Paul.

Soon after our move back, I began having problems with the unawareness of hypoglycemia. Every time I drove the car, I had to check my blood sugar before I started the engine. Before any public event, I had to check my blood sugar to see where I was. I checked my levels every two hours to save myself from accidents and embarrassment.

DeeDee was afraid to leave me alone, fearing I would run low and have problems. I assured her that I could handle this problem and attempted to do my best to keep my blood glucose between one hundred and two hundred, just to be safe.

For the next year or two, it was a juggling act of keeping a close eye on my every move and action. It was becoming frustrating. Each time I second-guessed myself, DeeDee was quick to ask, "What's your blood sugar?"

After many months of this problem, I asked friends if they could recommend a specialist in diabetes care. Remember, I had been a brittle diabetic for the past thirty years. The medical doctors tried me on different insulins made from beef, pork, and, in the end, genetic insulin. None of these types made much of a difference in my body.

Absorption seemed to be the main issue in my body, along with the beta cells. It appears that the beta cells in your bloodstream latch onto the insulin, and then they get absorbed into the blood, reducing the need for more insulin. The beta cells act like velcro, latching onto the insulin. However, after many years, they become worn out and lose the ability to latch onto the insulin, making it difficult to absorb into the bloodstream.

I was doing my best to handle the troubles, keeping a positive attitude toward the disease that was now rearing its ugly head in our lives! DeeDee was growing more frustrated with my medical problems. We had never had to deal with this issue before; it was a big obstacle in our everyday lifestyle.

On the day of Alanna's wedding, I was struggling to keep my blood glucose under control. I was officiating the ceremony and setting up for the reception that followed. I was checking my blood sugars and injecting insulin all day long. The wedding day went from early in the morning until late in the evening. I did not want to cause embarrassment for our family on the happiest day of her life. When all of the activities from the day ended, I returned late that evening, sat down in the chair in the living room, and passed out from exhaustion.

After the celebration of Derek and Alanna's wedding, I realized that I had to do something to make my health concerns easier to live with. DeeDee and I began searching for a specialist who would be able to help me with some of the complications from this disease.

I was determined to find a solution for my health problems and wanted only to find a specialist who could help me. I visited with two or three diabetes specialists, but I was not impressed with their knowledge or determination to solve problems. Most would simply say to me, "You are living with a disease that has no cure. There are only treatments for the disease."

I was a little disappointed with these specialists. I always thought that doctors helped fix things that were wrong with your body. How had they not found a cure yet? What were they waiting for? What about all of the new technology available? I had many questions and few answers at this point. I was growing weary over the deaths of loved ones and friends.

We eventually found a diabetes specialist in St. Paul, who came to me through many good recommendations. At our first meeting, the doctor listened to my health history with great interest and wanted to help with hypoglycemia unawareness. The doctor instructed me to continue with the frequent blood glucose testing. He suggested that I continue testing every two hours (and before driving a vehicle), faxing his office my blood test results on a weekly basis.

After a week or two of following his orders, he would make an insulin dosage change of one or two units. For five or six months, we went back and forth, and it was of no help to me. After six or seven months, I met with the doctor again and asked him, "Doc, how many patients do you treat with unawareness of hypoglycemia?" He responded, "One. You are my only patient with this complication."

Now I knew what I was up against. I was working with a practicing physician, and he was practicing on me. He had no experience with the complications that I was dealing with in my life! DeeDee and I continued to search for specialists who had experience treating hypoglycemia unawareness.

I was growing worse each and every month. I could not even trust myself any longer with this disease—it had taken over my life completely. Each and every time I left the house, I had a specific routine that I had to follow simply to travel and be safe in public.

After many conversations with medical doctors, we knew there had to be a solution. DeeDee did not give up researching the topic and talking with people. This was her starting point for patient advocacy! Frustration, information, and determination were the driving forces for DeeDee to help people with similar complications from the disease.

I visited with a new endocrinologist at an Allina Clinic. She had completed her medical school, internship, and fellowship training, so she was up to date with all of the current information on diabetes care. The problem was that she had very little experience with diabetics, except for newly diagnosed patients with the disease. She had no experience with those suffering from hypoglycemia unawareness.

After many visits with doctors and nurses under our belt, we attempted to find the best possible solution for the complications of the disease. DeeDee was the best person I could have in my corner. She loved talking on the telephone and finding solutions to problems. *My wish for every husband is to have a wife like mine!*

I needed help from above. We could not find a doctor who had experience. Many of the people we visited wanted to help us, but they simply couldn't without more experience.

With all of our efforts to find a specialist who could help us, I was growing very weary. Then it hit me! I had forgotten to go to the specialist of all specialists: the great physician, Jesus Christ! He has more knowledge about our bodies than anyone on earth. After all, He created all of us in His own image (Genesis 1:27).

Yes, sometimes, in our desperation to find someone to help us, we forget to go to our source and leave it in God's hands.

CHAPTER 6
THE UNIVERSITY OF MINNESOTA

"I pray that you may enjoy good health and that all may go well with you."
(3 John 2 NIV)

Hypoglycemia unawareness was a real complication in my life while living with Type 1. I sought out specialists to help me deal with the issues at hand, but to no avail. They were of no help to me.

After living with this complication for more than nine months, DeeDee called the University of Minnesota Hospital (U of M). She found out that the hospital was the major training center for pancreatic transplant surgeons. Dr. David Sutherland was one of the doctors present in 1966 at the first pancreas transplant in the world.

When DeeDee informed the lady on the telephone of my condition and how I had lived with the disease for more than thirty years, an appointment was made for me to be screened for a pancreas transplant. This was the only option for me.

My first appointment with the transplant team was on Shanna's birthday, August 3. We arrived back in Minnesota on August 2 after flying down to Florida to help drive our moving truck and minivan back to Minnesota.

The next morning, I went for my evaluation, screening, and testing for the transplant. This was a three-day event. After meeting with my pre-transplant coordinator, Marci Siers, I went through blood draws, physical examinations, and mental health evaluations. They check on you for everything. They do not want to waste a donor organ on someone who is not stable or well enough to receive the organ or graft.

I met with transplant surgeons, physician assistants, registered nurses, social workers, laboratory technicians, and others on the transplant team. I was blown away with the details involved in an organ transplant. The team checks you for everything: hepatitis A, B, and C; HIV/AIDS; sexually transmitted diseases; cancer; blood disorders; and liver, lung, and kidney functions. They also cross and type your blood for the future.

I had never given so many samples to any doctor before this. I had x-rays and ultrasounds of every part of my body. If you want to know what is going on with your body, sign up for a transplant evaluation!

After meeting with the transplant team for those three days and having all of the tests and samples given to the laboratory, I was told that I needed to see a heart physician for their clearance to move forward in the process.

After living with the disease for so many years, they needed to know if I had heart problems that needed to be dealt with before moving onto the transplant waiting list. Even though I told them that I had never had a problem with my heart and that it was in good shape, they would not listen to me. I was told to contact them after the heart surgeon cleared me to move forward.

I was a little put off by this. I had never been to see a heart surgeon before this evaluation. *How would they know what is going on with my heart anyway?*

Despite this, I worked at keeping a very good attitude with the transplant team. I wanted to set a good example of a believer in Christ. "Please" and "thank you" were used several hundred times while with the team. I put a smile on my face, asked many questions, and took meticulous notes from each of the many daily meetings. I felt very comfortable with the evaluation. Marci gave me several names to contact, all of whom received a pancreas or kidney transplant.

I called everyone on the list, asking them about the surgery and follow-up care. It was fun talking with people who had been given a second chance at life. Each and every person on the list was very thankful for the hospital, along with the skilled doctors and nurses who cared for them.

I found out that heart transplants are the easiest to perform; the doctor only needs to be a good plumber. Kidneys are also simple, relatively speaking, with many kidney transplants performed each week. However, pancreatic and intestinal transplants can be the most difficult to perform. The pancreas is an organ that sits behind the stomach and intestines. It does not like to be seen or touched. When the organ is taken from the donor body, it is handled by hand and becomes very irritated. It wants to be left alone, not seen or touched. Did you know that God made a glove compartment in your body? This open area is on the right-hand side of your abdomen, specifically made for spare parts (like organs) to fit in.

A person can now be a living donor by donating a kidney, up to half of their pancreas, or half of their liver. A liver will grow back to one hundred percent after nine or ten months. A single deceased organ donor can give their heart, lungs, kidneys, liver, pancreas, small and large intestines, eyes, tissue, and arteries. When a person is declared brain dead, they can help more than twelve people with a single donation. More about all of this later!

After visiting with the patients from the list that Marci gave me and reviewing my notes, I had many more questions to ask, but these would have to wait.

I made an appointment with Dr. Carmelo Pannetta, a heart surgeon at the University of Minnesota. After I arrived at Dr. Pannetta's office for my appointment, I asked him, "Why do you think I have a heart problem?"

He went on to say, "After living with the disease of diabetes for thirty-plus years, I know from experience that you will have heart problems. How would you like for the transplant team to stop your organ transplant, only to call me in to take over because you are having a heart attack? We need to deal with this before moving forward on the recipient transplant waiting list." That reasoning was good enough for me!

Dr. Pannetta discovered, after examining me and testing my heart with an EKG and stress test, that I had a bad lower anterior descending artery (LAD). He would need to do an angioplasty surgery and insert a stent. This surgery was scheduled a month out and we began to pray again. I had never had a single surgery in my lifetime. I needed a little help from the great physician, Jesus!

The month went by very quickly, and soon it was time for me to be admitted into the hospital for the surgery and a day of observation after the procedure.

I remember walking into the hospital and registering in the admission room. After this, I greeted the receptionist, Deb. I had known Deb for several years because I visited with patients at the hospital and would always greet her. She gave me free ministerial parking passes whenever I visited patients.

When Deb asked me who I was visiting today, I told her

that I was there for a minor surgery. She was shocked! I was very positive with her and always complimented her on her wonderful smile and pleasant personality. I thanked her after each and every visit for her help.

DeeDee and I walked down to the pre-surgery room to get prepared. Soon, Dr. Pannetta appeared. "Are you ready, Carl?" I replied back, "I'm ready if you are!"

I gave DeeDee a kiss, telling her that I loved her very much, and then I was rolled into the cath lab. I had never seen an operating room before and was amazed by all of the technology. There were giant monitor screens and lots of bright lights. One of the medical technicians asked me what type of music I wanted to listen to. I think I said jazz!

I was awake during the whole procedure, viewing the surgery on the giant monitors. I watched as Dr. Panetta inflated the balloon and installed the stents in my artery. He did fine work, and everything looked very good. He also installed a clamp on my groin to stop the bleeding. I was then rolled up to the heart floor of the hospital, where the nurses and medical staff took good care of me.

They monitored me for twenty-four hours. After this, I was released to go home and rest. Everything felt great, and I, along with DeeDee, were very happy to have this part of the evaluation completed.

After a week, I returned to Dr. Panetta's office for a follow-up visit. Dr. Panetta and DeeDee talked about their Italian families, laughing and joking around as if they had known each other for years. After examining me, the doctor scheduled a stress test for me again in three weeks. Before then, I was back at the doctor. This time, however, it was because I was having a heart attack! Dr. Panetta scheduled a surgery for me that day, so I was prepped for angioplasty surgery again.

Dr. Panetta found that the LAD had collapsed further

downline. He had to install more stents to strengthen and reinforce the artery so it could stay open. I was told that I had coronary heart disease. I would have to follow up with him yearly with EKGs and stress tests.

After another twenty-four hours of observation in the hospital, I was released and went home to rest. A week later, I returned to the doctor's office and was tested. Dr. Panetta gave me the okay to move forward with the transplant team. It was getting serious and a bit scary, but I continued to pray and believe. I was learning to walk by faith and not by sight.

CHAPTER 7
CONCERNED BUT NOT WORRIED

"Cast all your anxiety on Him because he cares for you."
(1 Peter 5:7 NIV)

I was cleared by Dr. Panetta to move forward with the transplant team in my evaluation. Two months have gone by since I spoke with my pre-transplant coordinator, Marci Siers, so I decided to check with her to see if she was going to list my name on the transplant waiting list.

However, Marci had some news she wanted to tell me. It turned out that the stool sample I submitted to the lab had come back with a large amount of blood showing up in it. She informed me that the doctors suspected I had colon cancer. They were confident I needed to be treated and cleared of cancer before getting on the list. The first step in the process was taking a colonoscopy, which I said I would do as soon as possible.

On the drive home from the hospital, I prayed and asked God for help again. When DeeDee arrived home from work, I explained to her the new obstacle in our way. We prayed together and left it in God's hands. The big thing I was dealing with was inside my head. Oh, how the devil plays with our minds. He is like a roaring lion who seeks to devour and destroy (1 Peter 5:8).

DeeDee called the hospital and made an appointment for me to have a colonoscopy in five days. The doctor performing the procedure informed me that he would be searching for polyps and removing them, as well as looking for cancer cells and removing those for a biopsy to be performed by the laboratory.

When I was taken into the procedure room, I was greeted by a friendly group of doctors, nurses, and medical technicians. The nurse instructed me to lie down on the table and get comfortable as the doctor explained the procedure he would follow in my body. Afterwards, he asked if I was ready, to which I replied, "Yes, let's get this chicken kicking!"

I watched as the camera slowly traveled through my colon. It was very interesting to me, as I had never seen the inside of my colon before. It appeared that the cleansing part of the colonoscopy was good; it was as clean as a whistle inside.

The doctor found a small polyp and quickly snipped it with his device, sending it off for a biopsy. There were no other spots that looked like cancer cells. The physicians believed that I was filled with cancer in my colon, but I believe that God healed me in answer to our prayers and for His glory and honor! To God be the glory forever!

The doctor removed the scope and finished the procedure. I thanked everyone in the room for doing such an outstanding job and asked them to forward the results of the colonoscopy to the transplant team, along with the biopsy information.

From there, they asked me to enter the "gas room." After colonoscopies are completed, everyone is told to lie down in this room on a bed and rest for an hour or two. There are multiple beds in the room, with only a fabric curtain separating them. I guess it was for privacy; however, it didn't work too well. You could hear everything in the room.

I would not like to be the nurse assigned to this room. This lady was a real champion. She encouraged the people in the room to have "air releases" from the gas or air that was forced into the colon during the colonoscopy. When I arrived in the room and laid down on the bed, the nurse introduced herself and encouraged me to "let it all out."

There were two or three other people in the room with me. The nurse was really excited about the older lady in the bed next to mine. She must have really had a lot of air inside her colon because she had some very loud and long toots! Each time I heard an "air release," the nurse would clap from the other side of the curtain and say, "That was a good one; good for you! Can you do more? Oh good. There's another one. You're doing so great! Can you give me one more? Oh, that's a good one too!"

The nurse was really an encourager. I do not know how she did that day after day. She did seem to enjoy her work, though! God bless her!

The older lady next to me should have gotten an award or two for the loudest and most frequent "air releases." I did not think ladies had those kinds of sounds coming out of their bodies.

After this experience was over, I drove the car home, laughing the entire time. I can only imagine what people driving past me thought I was listening to in my car. When DeeDee arrived home from work, we laughed about my experience and thanked God for healing my body again. To God be the glory forever!

Marci called me a few days later to tell me that she was waiting for some additional paperwork to arrive for her files.

Finally, it looked as though every step had been taken to move forward.

I was once again cleared by my gastroenterologist, who confirmed that I did not have colon cancer or anything else wrong. I was ready to move forward again with the transplant team. Six months had gone by since I began the evaluation process.

Marci reviewed all of my test results and was waiting on some additional paperwork to be processed by our health insurance company. DeeDee's health insurance was easy to work with, and they agreed to pay for everything required for the pancreas transplant. They were a bit slow with the paperwork but followed through with everything we desired.

They only add people to the National Transplant Waiting List twice a month, on the fifteenth and thirtieth. January 15 had slipped by us while we were waiting on the paperwork, but January 30 was approaching fast.

Marci called me on January 28 to inform me that she was adding my name to the waiting list early. The thirtieth was on a Sunday, so my name would be added to the list on January 28, 2004.

I was told to carry my cell phone with me twenty-four hours a day. A call could come at any time, day or night, informing me of an organ donation available for me. Each individual has the option to pass on an organ donation if they wish. I had my list of questions for the doctor when they called me folded up inside my wallet. All of these questions were important to me. I wanted to be as informed as I could before making a big decision about the transplant surgery needed to improve my life.

On Sunday morning, two days later, DeeDee and I were at Cedar Valley Church attending service when my cell phone vibrated during the worship service. I quickly looked down at the screen at the caller, who was from the hospital. I quickly walked outside of the sanctuary and answered the telephone, but it was the wrong number!

I believe it was God checking on me to make sure that I was ready for the actual call, which was coming sooner than I thought or expected.

Our hope and prayers were for the timing to be perfect in both the donor's life and ours. It is a very big deal when you are waiting for someone to die so that you can get a second chance at life on this earth. DeeDee and I prayed over this decision many times. When the call came, I wanted to be ready and informed on everything needed for the transplant surgery to be blessed by God!

I had spent six months with the transplant team and the evaluation process. I had been tested and retested for every kind of health problem in this world! I had received two heart angioplasty surgeries and suffered one heart attack, and I had beaten the colon cancer that the doctors were positive I had. We were now as ready as possible for the answer to our prayers!

CHAPTER 8
THREE DAYS LATER

"Therefore, if anyone is in Christ, the new creation has come: The old has gone, the new is here!"
(2 Corinthians 5:17 NIV)

Three days later, on February 3, 2004, I was working on my computer in our home office when my cell phone rang—only three days after being added to the list!

I answered the telephone, and a male voice asked, "Am I talking with Carl? This is Dr. Kandaswamy. I have a pancreas for you from a brain-dead donor."

I began asking the doctor my list of questions.

"Was the donor in a motor vehicle accident?"

"Yes. A single vehicle accident."

"Did the donor have any abdominal injuries in the accident?"

"No. Only head and brain trauma."

"How old is the donor?"

"He is twenty-one years old."

"Is the donor of average weight?"

"Yes. He has a very low body fat ratio and has a very athletic body."

"Where is the donor now? How close is he to the hospital?"

"He is in a local hospital. We have a transplant team on the way to the hospital now to harvest his organs."

I asked the doctor about the antigen match and the blood tests that were drawn from the donor. Dr. Kandaswamy responded to my questions with a shorter amount of patience. "Carl, the tests have all come back very positive. We have found nothing in his blood. You are a near-perfect match. Are you healthy? Do you have a cold or a fever?"

"No, I am not sick," I responded. "And, yes, I want the donor organ!"

He asked how quickly I could arrive at the hospital, to which I responded that I could be there in two hours. "Very good," he said. "Check in, and we will get ready for your transplant surgery now."

I called my wonderful wife, DeeDee, and gave her the news, asking her to come home from work early to pick me up and bring me to the hospital. I then paused, kneeled down by my office chair, and thanked God for my donor's life. I prayed for the family members who were grieving the death of their twenty-one-year-old son, grandson, brother, cousin, friend, and loved one. I wept out loud for his family and asked God to send the Holy Spirit to be their comforter in this difficult time period of his final minutes of breath on this earth.

DeeDee picked me up at home, we loaded our hospital bags (which we had packed in advance) into the car, and we began the hour-long drive to the hospital. DeeDee and I talked about the conversation I had with Dr. Kandaswamy about the transplant surgery and prayed together for the donor family and my surgery.

After checking in at the registration desk, we were told to go to the transplant floor to check in with my nurse, Rita, who was waiting for me. DeeDee and I rode the elevator up and walked quickly to the transplant wing of the hospital. We checked in at the nurse's desk and were told to go to our room.

My nurse, Rita, came to my hospital room to inform us of the procedure that would take place before the transplant surgery. They rolled me to the pre-op surgery floor as DeeDee walked beside my bed, holding my hand and praying for me.

I remember the pre-op nurse and the anesthesiologist asking me questions and telling me that they would be with me during the twelve-plus hour surgery. The anesthesiologist then told me that he would put me to sleep so the team of doctors and nurses could prepare my body for the surgery since the donor's pancreas had arrived at the hospital.

I gave DeeDee a kiss, telling her that I loved her and would see her smiling face in a few hours. A mask was then put over my face, and I was told to count backwards from ten to one.

I remember counting down slowly. *Ten, nine, eight, seven, six, five, four...* and I was out! The next thing I saw was the smiling, friendly face of a nurse in the recovery room. She asked me how I felt, and I told her I was a little groggy.

The nurse told me I had gone through a twelve-hour surgery and that they had to replace all of the blood in my body during it. She explained that I would be a little sore and that they would move me to the transplant floor after I regained some more strength and awoke from the effects of the anesthesia drugs.

I fell back asleep and was awakened by DeeDee's voice. She told me she loved me and told me how good I looked... She lied! I did not look good, but I knew she loved me.

When I arrived back at the transplant floor, Rita had gone

home from her shift, so I was taken care of in the morning by a fabulous nurse named Katie Huseth. Katie had a smile that lit up the room and had a very caring, lovely voice. She spoke confidently as she explained what she was doing for me in detail.

Later that morning, I felt more awake and was able to talk with DeeDee, asking her to call Dr. Panetta's office and inform him of my transplant surgery. She called him, and he stopped by to visit us in my hospital room a little later that day. Dr. Panetta was very happy for us and asked if he could check my blood levels on the computer in my room. After some checking and reading the blood tests and levels, he walked away from the computer screen, telling us, "I have some bad news for you. Your troponin level is bad; you're having a heart attack right now!"

Dr. Panetta left my room to meet with the transplant team. After a few minutes, he returned, informing me that I was going in for heart surgery. My nurse, Katie, prepared my body for the quick surgery, and within minutes, the transport people wheeled my bed down to the cath lab. I kissed DeeDee goodbye, told her I loved her, and got prepared for angioplasty surgery. Again.

I was awake for the surgery and was aware of the attention everyone gave to it. It was not business as usual. After Dr. Panetta finished lining my LAD with stents, he installed a clamp on my wrist to stop the bleeding from the artery. I was returned to the heart floor, not the transplant floor, for observation and follow-up. I had a great nurse, but she was not knowledgeable about transplant care.

The clamp had to be loosened a quarter turn every thirty minutes, like the groin clamp. When my nurse on the heart floor looked at the clamp, she said to me, "I have never seen one of these before." She looked at it, turning the knob to loosen it. When she did this, it fell off my wrist and onto the floor. She quickly picked it up from the floor, trying to reattach it, but she couldn't!

Since I was feeling fine and wasn't bleeding out, she kept an eye on my wrist, feeling it every thirty minutes, until I was transferred back to the transplant floor the next day. It felt good to get back where I belonged!

I asked DeeDee to check the Minneapolis Star Tribune newspaper for the obituary notice of a twenty-one-year-old male. As she showed me a picture and obituary for Grant Glazier, the Holy Spirit showed me that he was my donor. I told her to save that page from the newspaper for me to read and use later before we once again prayed for the Glaziers!

The new pancreas was performing well, and the anti-rejection drugs were too. Everything was going well, and after seven days on the transplant floor, the doctors were ready to release me in a few more days.

Our oldest granddaughter, Blake Madison, was celebrating her sixth birthday on February 10. We celebrated her at the hospital, and on Valentine's Day, she handed out candy to the transplant staff, nurses, and aides—they loved it!

I noticed this and told DeeDee that we needed to provide a candy dish for the nurses and staff. They were so busy and had no time to eat—they needed a little pick-me-up during their shifts. This is how we started sharing candy with the hospital. When the staff at the hospital saw the candy dish, they would know I was admitted to the hospital again.

Everyone watched my labs closely and continued to monitor me with great attention and care. I was struggling with extreme pain and infections that seemed to linger in my body.

After two weeks in the hospital, I was talking with my father over the telephone when he told me that he, my brother Tom, and my sister Linda were allergic to morphine, which is used to kill pain. DeeDee quickly shared this information with the medical staff and doctors, who stopped the drug and switched me to the painkiller dilaudid.

Within days, I started to feel better. I was no longer nauseated and throwing up, my fever reduced, and it appeared like I was getting ready to go home again. I had two or three good days and was keeping food down. I had a great nurse, Tony Sioco, who understood what it was like for transplant patients. They had removed over fourteen feet of my intestines during the surgery to connect the drainage for the pancreas into my body, as it is the natural way for drainage.

After a few more minor setbacks in the hospital, it had now been thirty days since I was admitted. The average stay for a pancreas transplant was ten to fourteen days, so I was more than double the average. DeeDee never left my side and slept in the room with me in every kind of chair, lounger, cot, or window sill and in every kind of sleeping position possible. She found places to shower, change, and even wash her clothes. My mother was also a big help to us, along with our children and grandchildren.

We built great relationships with the doctors, nurses, aides, lab techs, and other medical staff members. I was familiar with the radiologists, the ultrasound personnel, the people from transport, and all of the transplant team.

When the doctors finally felt comfortable enough to discharge me from the hospital in early March, it took hours to say goodbye to everyone, thanking them for all of their help! I was finally able to go home and start recovering from my multiple surgeries over the past month.

CHAPTER 9
TWENTY-SEVEN MONTHS OF A NEW LIFE

"I know, O LORD, that the way of man is not in himself, that it is not in man who walks to direct his steps."
(Jeremiah 10:23 ESV)

On March 8, 2014, I had a follow-up doctor's appointment with Dr. Kandaswamy. He checked my blood for indicators of the pancreas graft. Everything seemed to be working great, and he explained to me that I would need to have my blood drawn twice a week for a few months. My post-transplant coordinator, Maureen, would keep a close eye on my numbers.

I went home from the doctor's office feeling great. For the first time in over thirty years, I was able to have "my birthday cake and eat it too!" I could eat as much cake and ice cream as I wanted with no effect on my blood glucose.

I was having a barbecue outside, and as I set up the picnic table on this beautiful spring day, our daughter Shanna arrived with the grandkids for my birthday party. Shanna noticed I was drinking a Sprite. She said, "Dad! You're not drinking Diet Coke! That's a regular Sprite; it isn't sugar-free!" "It's all right!" I responded. "I can drink and eat anything that I want now!"

The U of M transplant team made each of the transplant recipients responsible for calling in their blood test results and knowing the names and doses of the prescription drugs they were taking multiple times per day. After I called the transplant team and told them my numbers, my coordinator would call me back to advise on any changes needed for the remainder of the week.

The most important information they wanted were the amylase and lipase levels from the blood draws. The levels for hemoglobin, creatinine, white and red blood cell counts, and glucose were also important to note. Maureen did a great job using this information to discuss my transplant with the transplant team.

I was enjoying a new life with my nearly new pancreas—it was only twenty-one years old and was working great for me. Thank you, Grant. You were a giver in life and in death!

I wrote a letter to the donor family; however, it could not include last names or locations. It had to be generic in flavor. If LifeSource, the donor agency, thought the letter was too personal, they would mark parts of it out with a thick, black marker. I wrote the letter with this in mind.

It took the agency a month or so to read my letter and forward it to the Glazier family. Only ten to fifteen percent of patients ever write a thank you letter or send a card to a donor family, and very few family members ever write back to the recipient. What a shame!

After five or six weeks, I received an envelope in the mail from LifeSource that included a letter from Grant's mother, Connie. The letter confirmed everything that God revealed to me earlier. The last names were marked out, along with some other information.

In the letter from Connie Glazier, she described her son

Grant. He was a six-foot-eight-inch, two-hundred-pound basketball and football star from Annandale High School who went on to play basketball and football in college. He had hundreds of friends and around forty or fifty close friends. He watched the Sunday evening Super Bowl game with many of his friends on the night he was in his car accident.

It had snowed and the roads were icy when Grant was driving home from the Super Bowl party. His car started to spin on the icy roadway, crashing into a pickup truck. Grant was taken to St. Cloud Hospital by ambulance, where they ran tests on his brain and discovered that he was brain dead —there was no brain activity or blood flow to the brain. Grant's only injuries from the car accident were to his brain; the rest of his body was unharmed.

Grant died from his injuries fifteen hours later, on Monday, February 2, 2004. He was kept alive only by the respirator and life support equipment until his organs could be harvested and used to give life or improve life for others.

It was only a short time before the hospital staff asked Connie if she wanted to donate Grant's organs to people in need. At first, Connie said no because she was still in shock over her son's death. After a few hours, though, Connie changed her mind. "Grant was a giver in life. He would be a giver in death also," she said. She then returned to the hospital with her family to say goodbye to Grant.

I called LifeSource and sent in a form to release my personal information to Grant's family. They forwarded a form to Connie, asking if she wanted to contact me without them in the middle, which she agreed to. Within a month or so, we received each other's information, so I picked up the telephone and called her. We talked for an hour or more, and I expressed how thankful DeeDee and I were for Grant's pancreas in my body!

We set up a time to meet the family and friends of Grant at

the Glazier's home. Two newspapers were there, the St. Cloud Times and the Annandale Advocate, along with two television stations that recorded our meeting and interviewed us for their 10:00 p.m. news broadcast. Our story led the news program for WCCO Channel 4, CBS, and KARE 11 (the NBC affiliates in the Twin Cities).

DeeDee and I met Grant's family members and over one hundred of his friends at his family's home in Annandale. DeeDee and I stayed connected with them. There's no way I would be alive and doing well without this gift. Being thankful for Grant's gift of life seemed like the right thing to do!

Grant's pancreas gave me a second chance at living a great life without complications from the disease without a cure. It felt great! I continued with my blood draws and often went to the procedure room at the transplant center for a drug called ChemPath. This anti-rejection drug was used to treat the blood cells, which attacked the pancreas graft because it was a foreign object in my body.

I had thirteen ChemPath treatments in my body until the FDA pulled it from the marketplace because too many people were dying from the drug. While it helped me, it killed many people in treatment.

Since I was feeling great, I decided to return to the ministry. DeeDee and I were approached by a pastor friend of ours, Pastor Denny Curran, from Cold Spring, Minnesota, to start a new church in the city of Sartell. This was located in the middle of the state, an hour and twenty minutes from Minneapolis-St. Paul.

We planned the grand opening of the new church for Sunday, November 11, 2004. I had visited three Lutheran churches, a Catholic church, and a Presbyterian church in the area. We also attended each one of their Sunday morning worship services, informing the pastors that we were opening a Pentecostal, Charismatic, Full Gospel church in town with the aim of loving and discipling the community in the name of the Lord Jesus Christ.

I had done my homework on the city—five Full Gospel, Charismatic churches had opened in the city within the last eight years. None of them lasted more than nine months before closing the doors. This county had the largest number of Roman Catholics per capita of any other, second only to Rome, Italy.

There was a religious spirit in the city that needed to be broken, and I knew it would only happen through prayer and fasting. I had never been able to fast before receiving the pancreas transplant, but now I was ready! I started a forty-day fast and prayer for our church and to break down the religious spirit in the city. My fasting ended with our grand opening.

After we opened, I was attacked by the religious spirit in my body. I had very bad pain in my abdomen area. I knew where the pain was coming from and why I was being attacked for my faith.

I went to my transplant doctor, Dr. Sutherland, who, after examining me, ordered ultrasounds, x-rays, and MRIs. It looked like I had pancreatitis, which is only cured by removing the pancreas when the pain becomes unbearable. I had only had the pancreas for one year. It was working fine, but the pain was very, very difficult to endure. We prayed, but nothing seemed to help me.

I could not keep food down any longer and had to use total parenteral nutrition (TPN) twenty-four hours a day. I carried a bag of fluid nutrition everywhere I went. It was my only hope; the pain was growing worse each and every day.

We prayed and believed God for a miracle, casting the religious spirit out many times. Yet the pain and hospitalizations became more frequent. After ten months of extreme pain, I asked Dr. Sutherland to remove the pancreas graft, making sure he harvested the islet cells from the pancreas and injected them into the portal vein to my liver.

Dr. Sutherland had performed many islet cell transplants, but I was the first allot islet cell transplant from a donor graft organ. We had extreme faith and knew that my islet cells were producing more than enough insulin for my body to use—Dr. Sutherland simply had to harvest them, inject them into my liver, and let them find a home to grow and work for me.

I had a twenty-two-month vacation from the disease with no cure. I was insulin-free and had no finger pricks during that time. I had no restrictions on my diet and lived life to the fullest. I was so thankful and enjoyed every minute with the pancreas graft from Grant Glazier!

DeeDee and I arrived at the hospital and checked in for my surgery. We met with Dr. Sutherland in the pre-op room, where he briefed us on how he would perform the surgery and the steps he would take to make it successful. The anesthesiologist also came in to explain how he would put me to sleep for the surgery so I would not feel anything. I said goodbye to DeeDee, kissing her on the forehead and telling her that I loved her and would see her smiling face later!

The anesthesiologist covered my mouth with a mask, and I counted backwards. *Ten, nine, eight, seven...* and I was out cold.

When Dr. Sutherland opened my incision again for the third time, he saw that there was only a small portion of the pancreas graft that looked bad. While he thought about simply removing that bad portion of the pancreas and leaving it alone, he still removed the graft and began harvesting the islet cells from it. He was able to harvest more than enough cells from the graft and inject more than enough of them into the portal vein of my liver. He cleaned up my abdominal area and closed the incision, completing the surgery in about four hours.

Transport wheeled the bed back to the transplant floor, where my transplant nurses took great care of me as I rested the remainder of the day. DeeDee sat beside my bed the entire day, waiting for me to wake up and talk with her.

Late in the afternoon, Dr. Sutherland stopped by the room to check on my condition. He informed DeeDee and I that the surgery went well—now it was up to those islet cells to find a home in my liver and go to work for my body. The lab techs continued to check my blood every four to six hours, and the nurses would check my glucose every two hours. This was the sign we were looking for to know if the cells would work.

After patiently waiting two or three days, Dr. Sutherland explained that things were not looking good for me. It appeared that the cells were not working in my liver. We would give it another five to seven days, but I needed insulin injections starting that day. The transplant doctors, nurses, aides, lab techs, social workers, and transport were all concerned with how I was doing physically, mentally, and emotionally.

With DeeDee's help, we continued to be positive in every circumstance, believing that God had the best plan for my life. Many of our newfound friends at the hospital asked us, "How do you stay so positive and stop the depression in your lives?" My response was always the same: "How can I be depressed when I look at all that Jesus Christ has done for me on the Cross of Calvary?"

We could always get a smile and a head nod from the people who asked me that question. More times than not, we built people up and encouraged them when they were there to encourage us!

After a twenty-seven-month vacation from diabetes, I walked out of the hospital as a Type 1 diabetic again. The transplant doctors had hoped that my body would reset and that I would not have the problem of hypoglycemia unaware-ness. However, this was not the case. I was now back with the same set of problems I had before the original transplant. DeeDee was not able to leave me alone while she went to work, so my mother came to our house and stayed with me while DeeDee was at work.

Physically, I was now back to where I was before. I was using the same treatment as before but with a completely different set of health issues, including an incision in my abdomen (from my groin to six inches below my breast) that would not heal and weak circulation in my legs that made the skin on both of my legs black.

My mother would attach pumps to each of my legs for ninety minutes a day per leg to help me with the lymphedema. A home care nurse visited me daily to install a wound VAC in my abdomen. For two and a half hours, the machine would help heal my incision.

My mother stayed very busy as she connected and discon-nected machines to my legs and abdomen during the day. She also read healing scriptures over me by the hour every day to ease my pain.

It was hard for me to not be discouraged. The healing process was slow, but I was making small steps toward improvement. When you're in the biggest fight of faith you've ever faced, it's important that you resist the urge to not go by what you see.

Although healing was moving at a snail's pace, it was moving. Hallelujah! There are no shortcuts to waiting on God. Now was not the time to give up, so we kept trusting that I would get better.

CHAPTER 10
HOME CARE NURSES

"I was sick and you looked after me."
(Matthew 25:36 NIV)

DeeDee was advised by the social workers at the hospital to admit me into a nursing home or skilled care nursing facility, but she wanted nothing to do with this kind of care, so she learned the skills needed to care for me at our home. She did this with the help of a home care nurse named Karen Norgard, who worked for Northfield Home Care.

Karen was a very bright light on many of our darkest days. Karen's smile would make you happy, no matter how bad you felt. Her cheerful voice and quick-witted humor on her daily visits were the best parts of the day.

Nurse Karen would take my temperature, blood pressure, other vitals, and clean my unhealed incision area. She installed the wound VAC in my abdomen and inspected my legs for lymphedema. Twice a week, she would also draw my blood for testing.

When someone spends an hour or two with you daily, you

become close to each other. After two years, Karen, along with myself, my mother, and DeeDee, became close friends! We united around one cause: helping me become healthy and strong again. Karen was a lifesaver with her help on these daily visits. I always looked forward to them!

Frequently, once a month or so, I was admitted to the hospital for infections, lymphedema, fevers, and other medical health issues. My hospital stays were between five and seven days long and often included being given very strong IV antibiotics to stop the infections.

Any time my temperature went above one hundred degrees, I was told to report to the emergency room to be seen by a doctor. This usually meant another five- to seven-day hospital stay. My stays became so frequent that most of the doctors and nurses in the emergency department knew me by my first name and became very good friends with DeeDee.

We carried along in our hospital bags letters from my doctors that gave the emergency room doctors all of the information needed concerning my IV doses, pain medication, and other practical steps to take while I was in the emergency room, waiting for a room on the transplant floor. With each and every visit to the emergency room, we learned how to help them help me in a much more efficient manner. The goal of each hospitalization was to make it easier on everyone and to get admitted into a room on the transplant floor.

Karen was my home care nurse for two years until she was offered a new job and accepted it. On her last day, she called on me at our home and was very sad. Karen knew me better than anyone in my life. She helped with my health problems and issues and knew every part of my body in detail.

When she left, they sent another nurse over to the house,

who I had seen once or twice before while Karen was on vacation. The new nurse was Alison Valinski.

Alison was a very positive person with a great sense of humor, and within weeks, we became close. Alison enjoyed my mother, who was my personal care attendant (PCA). DeeDee also enjoyed the twice-a-week visits with Alison.

Alison was quick to take care of my needs and move on to the next patient due to her very busy days. Whenever she had to follow up with me later in the day to add TPA to my PICC line or fix a clog, she was efficient and always took the time necessary to help us understand what was going on inside my body.

A good-hearted welcome and a wonderful joke at the end of our home care visits always made the day easier to deal with. I am thankful for all the wonderful people that the Lord brought our way to be a part of our health care team. I realize that these relationships were God-ordained—a gift from Him. At home or at the hospital, Jesus was with me. It wasn't fun to walk through this, but He was my strength and my help, and He was in control. I had one job: *trust Him.*

CHAPTER 11
HEALTHY ENOUGH FOR A TRANSPLANT AGAIN

"Every good and perfect gift is from above, coming down from the Father of the heavenly lights, who does not change like shifting shadows."
(James 1:17 NIV)

I was in my home office on the morning of November 17, 2007, when our telephone rang. I answered the phone even though I did not recognize the voice on the other end of the line.

It was a female voice who said, "This is Dr. Ty Dunn, from the University of Minnesota Transplant Center. Are you healthy, Carl?" I answered Dr. Dunn with one word: "YES!" She continued, "I have a donor pancreas available for you. Are you interested?"

I was not prepared to answer this type of question. It came as kind of a shock to me—I did not remember going back on the transplant waiting list.

After several seconds of time (even though it seemed like hours to me), I began to understand what Dr. Dunn was talking with me about. I looked through my wallet, looking for my old question list for the doctor, but I couldn't find it, so I asked the questions that popped into my mind.

DeeDee walked into my home office midway through the conversation, and after hanging up the telephone with the doctor, we discussed the upcoming surgery, praying for the donor's family and the procedure. Within minutes, DeeDee loaded up our hospital bags into the car. We both frantically made calls to our loved ones, informing them of the transplant surgery and asking them to pray for the donor's family and myself.

While traveling to the hospital in the car, we talked on cell phones and prayed for all the upcoming events of the day ahead. The hour-long ride to the hospital went by so quickly. It was as if someone had the clock on fast-forward.

Upon our arrival at the hospital, I checked in at the registration desk and was told to go to the transplant floor to check in with my transplant nurse. All of the medical staff on the transplant floor were excited when they saw DeeDee and I arrive. They knew why we were there and could not wait for me to get into the pre-op room for surgery.

Soon, the physician assistant and my transplant nurse were asking me all of the questions necessary for the surgery and briefing me on all of the important information. The lab tests for my blood came back, and they were all negative—which is positive!

Transport arrived, ready to move me to the pre-op room for surgery. DeeDee and I waved to everyone on the floor as we left and told them we'd be back in twelve to fourteen hours.

The anesthesiologist came to me with a very large stack of paper, which were my medical records. After several minutes of reviewing them, the doctor explained the procedure and how she would be with me through the end of the surgery.

I was once again told to say goodbye to DeeDee. I gave

her a kiss, telling her that I loved her very much and was looking forward to seeing her in the recovery room in a few hours. I also told her not to have too good of a time in the waiting room! They then rolled my bed into the operating room and began the pancreas transplant surgery, which would last more than ten hours.

When I woke up in the recovery room, there was a wonderful nurse who told me the surgery went very well. They would soon get my wife for me, and, after an hour or two, they would move me back up to the transplant floor for post-surgery care.

When I saw DeeDee's smiling face and heard her comforting voice, I was overjoyed! She told me about all the fun they had in the waiting room during my surgery. This was becoming a habit for my family!

I fell asleep again while DeeDee talked with me. I was so tired, sleepy, and sore. After an hour or so, they moved me back to the transplant floor, and all of the transplant nurses wanted to care for me. It felt good seeing all of the familiar faces in my room—the nurses did a great job caring for me. The lab techs all knew me by name and drew my blood for the tests needed to review my numbers.

For the first day, I was in and out of sleep for most of the time. Dr. Dunn stopped by to see us and shared how the surgery went. Everything looked good, and she had put the drain from the pancreas graft into my intestines. She believed that the graft looked very healthy and would be a good organ for me. She also told us that she performed a little cosmetic surgery on my belly button to clean it up from past surgeries.

I asked her how my numbers looked, but she said that it was too soon to tell. The pancreas does not like to be seen, much less touched and transplanted, so she told us to give it some time to settle down.

The next day, Dr. Dunn stopped by the room in the

morning to follow up with me. I told her that something was wrong inside of me. She reviewed my labs and asked what it felt like. All I could tell her was that something was wrong. She immediately scheduled the operating room and told the nurses to prep me for surgery. The doctors here knew that I was not a complainer, so if I said something was wrong, something had to be wrong with me.

I was rushed into surgery and awoke several hours later in the recovery room, feeling totally different. The recovery nurse was pleasant but not talkative like in the previous surgeries I had been through. DeeDee was not her cheerful self either. That evening, Dr. Dunn stopped by the hospital room and updated us.

There was something wrong inside me, like I had felt. She explained that there was a blood clot that stopped the flow of blood to the pancreas graft, killing it. She had to remove the graft, making the transplant unsuccessful.

We thanked Dr. Dunn for her help and efforts, and then she left our room. The medical staff and nurses asked if we wanted to see a social worker to talk about it. We said no, and we continued to seek God for answers to our questions and to trust Him. We kept a positive attitude and tried to encourage others on the floor. We spent forty-seven days in the hospital.

It was different going home this time—I had gone through two very difficult surgeries. I left the hospital with nothing positive, just forty-seven days of pain, suffering, and infections. When DeeDee and I drove home, I don't think we said one word to each other the whole trip.

My nurse, Alison, was scheduled to see me the next day. I was very sore from the two incisions again—this was now the fifth time they had opened my abdomen up.

When Dr. Dunn opened me up for the emergency surgery to remove the graft, she was not able to save my belly button. She had to cut it out, which left an awful-looking scar and wasn't healing properly. Our grandsons, Gavin and Grady, told me, "PaPa, you will be easy to identify in Heaven! Only you and Adam won't have a belly button!"

Alison visited with us the next day to draw my labs and care for my incision. She was the only person who was not depressed, and it was an attitude that we appreciated! I knew thAt when I was healed, I wanted to be like Alison for others. I learned a lot from her about the power of a positive attitude.

CHAPTER 12
INFECTIONS AND MONTHLY HOSPITALIZATIONS

"But now, Lord, what do I look for? My hope is in you."
(Psalm 39:7 NIV)

After becoming a transplant recipient, you are required to take a prescribed drug called CellCept to lower your immune system. The immune system must be lowered because it identifies the transplanted graft as a foreign object, attacking the organ.

CellCept lowered my immune system but also lowered my white and red blood cell count. A normal person's red blood cell count is 4.32 to 5.73, but mine was 3.0. A normal person's white blood cell count is between 5.0 and 10.0, but my white blood cell count was 2.0 or less, which is more than half of what it should have been. When my white blood cell count would go up to between 3.0 and 4.0, the doctors knew my body was fighting an infection somewhere. This usually meant a hospital stay of five or seven days.

My platelet count was also very low. Platelets help to clot the blood or stop the blood from flowing when there is an injury. The average person's platelet count ranges between 150 and 450, but my average count was below 70.

I was given weekly Aranesp injections to help my body raise the hemoglobin in my blood. However, this was an expensive drug, and each weekly injection cost more than one thousand dollars.

The hospital checked my bone marrow, which produces the white blood cells. They inject a three- or four-inch needle into the base of your back, withdrawing a syringe of bone marrow to examine. The pain is excruciating when they withdraw the bone marrow from you. It is not a fun day! Upon examining my bone marrow, they could not figure out why my body was not producing more white blood cells. I had to go through this procedure twice.

In spite of all of the precautions taken, about once a month I was admitted to the hospital with an infection somewhere in my bloodstream.

In the hospital, the doctors would always want to remove my PICC line, thinking that it was the cause of the infection. After removing it from my arm and testing it in the lab, it would come back negative, which is a positive thing in the hospital world. The doctors would treat my blood infection with IV antibiotics, releasing me after installing a new PICC line in the upper part of my other arm.

The doctors discharged me and hoped for the best. DeeDee and my mother were very careful when they injected anything into the PICC line, and they cleaned it several times per day; however, the line was never the source of any infection.

My symptoms were always the same. I would become very nauseous and not be able to keep my oral pain medication down. My temperature would go up to one hundred degrees or more, which meant an automatic visit to the ER.

My body would become septic, and my organs would start shutting down—specifically my kidneys.

Many times, I was transported to the hospital by ambulance. Within three or four hours, my condition could change dramatically to the point where I needed the paramedics' help for the one-hour trip to the hospital. The Northfield Ambulance's paramedics knew me well and were very good at taking care of me on the trip to Minneapolis.

We would arrive at the emergency room with documents in hand to show the ER doctors, as well as documents for the physicians on other floors, when we could not get me into the transplant floor. And, of course, we brought bags of candy with us for the medical staff whenever we came.

DeeDee was great at calling the hospital and checking in with the transplant floor to find out the census and availability for my stay. Then, she would call patient placement to see where we could stay in the hospital. Being a frequent guest, you learned who and how to talk to different people to attain what you needed.

The doctors would give me IV antibiotics while in the hospital, and then would send me home with either the IV antibiotics or switch me to an oral antibiotic. DeeDee and my dear mother were very good at giving me IV antibiotics— both of them could have been nurses with the way they cared for me and gave me medications. They did this every two hours with such love and devotion.

Alison, my home care nurse, was always a joyful sight to see after my discharge from the hospital. She jumped right in with her sweet, wonderful care for me. Each time I would arrive home from the hospital, she would say, "You did it again; you are home! It's so good to have you back!"

However, the problem was that I didn't stay home for long. It seemed like my life had become trips to the ER—

staying in the hospital, only to come back home and repeat over and over again.

CHAPTER 13
THE DAY I DIED (THE FIRST TIME)

"Precious in the sight of the Lord is the death of His faithful servants."
(Psalm 116:15 NIV)

On November 17, 2008, one year to the date of my second solid organ transplant, I was preparing to go home after a hospital stay for another infection in my bloodstream. The doctors had removed my PICC line, which they thought was the source of the infection but wasn't. I needed a new PICC line installed in my arm for TPN. I had not eaten anything by mouth for almost two years.

DeeDee left me to go to work, and my mother was with me at the hospital. My transplant nurse for the day shift was Kate Remus. Transport came to my hospital room to take me down to vascular access, where they would install the new line before discharging me.

I said goodbye to my mother, telling her, "I will see you in a few minutes. I love you!" My mom had waited for me many times before when they installed new lines into my arm.

Mom was a professional at waiting for me to return and bringing me home from the hospital.

When I arrived at vascular access, Olga greeted me at the door and asked me to lie down on the table. She had installed lines in me fifteen or twenty times. She was a wonderful lady who was always cheerful and pleasant with me. Olga was installing a double lumen line, like so many other times; it was business as usual.

I laid down on the table as she gave me some novocaine to ease the pain, measured me for the line, and started inserting it into my vein. Everything was great, and it all seemed very normal.

After ten or fifteen minutes, the PICC line was in place and was tested with saline. I told her, "Thank you, Olga. You did a great job as always; I really appreciate you and thank you for your help." These were the last words I would speak...

Olga noticed I had stopped breathing, and she asked my nurse, Kate, if I was allergic to any new drugs. Kate told her to call the code!

I'm sure most of you have heard the code call over the PA system in the hospital. "Adult code blue vascular access" was repeated two or three times, alerting the cardiac arrest team to bring the crash cart and quickly report to the vascular access room. They run to the room and are prepared to go to work on you until your heart is beating again!

Kate ran to my hospital room and told my mother to hurry up and follow her. They ran down four flights of stairs to the vascular access room. When they got to the room, I was lying on the table with no movement. Olga had started CPR, and Kate took over until the crash cart personnel arrived within minutes.

The vascular access room was very small, and with the response team of four or five people, as well as Olga, Kate, and my mother in the room, it became very crowded. As the response team arrived, everyone else left the room. They stood in the hallway, looking through the doorway into the room, while the team worked to restart my heart.

My mother told me that when they paddled, shocked, or jump-started my heart, my legs and arms flew in the air. She described me as a fish out of water—flopping around like a fish on the dock, wanting to get back into the water.

The team jump started my heart three times. I was without a heartbeat for more than fifteen minutes. After the third time, the team was able to get a weak pulse, so they rushed me into the ICU, incubating me and hooking me up to life support equipment. I was attached to a respirator and heart machine with oxygen, and they gave me propofol, the drug Michael Jackson used to let him fall asleep (he called it "magic milk!").

My physician assistant called DeeDee on her cell phone at work, asking her to come back to the hospital as soon as possible. When she arrived at the ICU, she met my mother, and they came in to see me. I was in a coma, unable to do anything. My mother told DeeDee what happened and how everyone did everything possible as quickly as they could.

I was lifeless in the ICU for three days. DeeDee kept vigil for my healing while the doctors and medical staff continued to check for brain function and assess the damage and medical condition of my body.

DeeDee and I had discussed with each other years ago that neither of us wanted to be kept alive by machines. We wanted God to be in charge of our lives and our deaths. She knew all my desires, especially the fact that I did not want to be kept alive by a machine.

That small, quiet voice from Heaven spoke to her directly, telling her to disconnect me from life support. DeeDee waited three days and heard the audible voice from God!

She did not talk to my mother, our daughters, or anyone else. She asked to talk with the ICU doctors, telling them to disconnect me from life support. The doctors explained to her that I would die, but she told them, "We have talked about this for years. Carl does not want to be kept alive by a machine!" The doctors questioned her and asked if she wanted them to call someone for her, but she told them no.

The social workers and nurses, along with the doctors, tried to talk her out of the decision, but when you tell DeeDee your wishes, she sticks to them! I am thankful for her strong convictions and supernatural strength and faith.

After having her sign several documents advising her of her decision to disconnect life support for me, they went right to work. They closed the large glass doors, pulled the curtain, and disconnected me from the machine that was pumping my heart and breathing for me.

DeeDee said that I made a gurgling sound and tried to breathe—it sounded awful and strenuous—but after several minutes, I began to breathe somewhat normally. When the ICU doctor and nurse suctioned my throat and cleared the airway, I started breathing on my own.

We discovered later why my heart had stopped. On that day, my magnesium and potassium levels were at the low end of the normal scale. When Olga inserted the PICC line in my vein and got close to my heart, it must have tickled the heart and made it stop. From then on, a new blood test was given to me before a PICC line could be inserted. If my levels were not at the top of the normal scale, I was given more IV magnesium and potassium to raise them.

DeeDee found out years later that only ten percent of people live more than a year after being shocked back to life. They told us that I was very lucky. They say if your brain is without oxygen or blood flow for more than ten minutes, you experience brain damage. I tell people, "You will have to ask DeeDee if I have any brain damage because I cannot tell!"

A lot of people have asked me if I visited Heaven or hell when my heart stopped. I have to be honest with you; I did not visit either when I stopped breathing.

DeeDee and I have never feared death—our reservations are made and our names are written in the Lamb's Book of Life! When we die on this earth, all we have to do is "check-in" at the reservation desk at the pearly gates! Heaven is our life's reward!

I believe God knew that I was ready. I was already aware of both places: Heaven and hell. God knew I was going to live. He did not have to test me; it was all part of His glorious plan in my life that was dedicated to serving and living for Him.

I will never take life for granted again or live a day without giving thanks to my God for each and every moment that I can serve Him and others. Each day is a gift—that's why they call it the present!

CHAPTER 14
A MEDICAL TRIP TO IOWA

"But those who hope in the Lord will renew their strength. They will soar on wings like eagles; they will run and not grow weary, they will walk and not be faint."
(Isaiah 40:31 NIV)

I had a wonderful infectious disease doctor, Dr. JoAnne Young, who was concerned with the monthly infections in my body. Due to the many heavy-duty antibiotics used in the hospital and at home, she was worried they would stop working or my body would become immune to them. Dr. Young discussed this with DeeDee, asking her to do some research on the subject. The University of Minnesota was interested in hiring a specialist in this area of medicine but could not find a doctor willing to leave their practice.

DeeDee did her homework and discovered that within the local medical community and the Mayo Clinic in Rochester, Minnesota, no one had a specialist in this area of medicine. However, she did not take no for an answer! She found a wonderful and very successful doctor, Dr. Rao, who was a gastroenterologist at the University of Iowa. Iowa City, Iowa, was over two hundred and fifty miles from our home in Northfield, Minnesota.

After DeeDee talked with the doctor's nurse over the telephone, explaining my dilemma to her, the doctor was very interested in seeing me. He knew there was not a doctor like himself in the state of Minnesota—he had turned down the U of M several times over the past year or two to join them. DeeDee set up an appointment for me, which was difficult because he was so busy. He wanted me to stay for three days of testing.

Our next obstacle on this medical trip was traveling. I was very sick most of the time. I had not eaten any food for more than three years and had to be injected with IV Zofran every six hours to stop the nausea. I had to sleep in a recliner to keep my head raised, and my abdomen was in excruciating pain. I took pain medication every two hours, each and every day.

DeeDee and I knew that I could not fly to Iowa with all of my medical gear and TPN for three days. I became very ill simply by riding in a car for less than an hour twice a week, going back and forth to the hospital.

My wonderful, beautiful wife did what she always did over the years—she asked our home church to pray for us. The church prayed, and some wonderful friends of ours, Clyde and Karen Thompson, talked to DeeDee about the medical trip to Iowa.

Clyde and Karen used to travel to Arizona in the winter months to escape the cold Minnesota weather. This year, they were not traveling down to Arizona. Since their oldest son, Loren, and his wife, Shelly, owned a motorhome, Clyde and Karen were happy to drive us to Iowa City in it. They decided to vacation in the southern part of Iowa for three days with us.

This was an answer to our prayers. Clyde and Karen

picked us up at our home in Northfield on Sunday afternoon. The weather was cold, but the sun was shining and the roads were as clear as a July summer day. The motorhome was great to travel in for me. It had a restroom, and the seats were very comfortable and adjusted perfectly for me. Clyde was the perfect chauffeur, and Karen was the perfect hostess. I felt like I was traveling by air again, like air travel was in the 1960s.

We visited and got caught up on the Thompson family, sharing about our family too. It was a fun time: we laughed, told stories about our church memories, and enjoyed the beautiful small-town country scenery of Iowa as we traveled through the state.

I also made sure to tell as many jokes as I had about Iowa.

What's the best thing coming out of Iowa? *Interstate I-35 North!*

Why do they have AstroTurf at all of the football fields in Iowa? *To keep the cheerleaders from grazing!*

I would tell people from Iowa, "If you place your Iowa driver's license on the dashboard of your car, you can park in any handicapped space!" However, after our medical trip to Iowa, I stopped telling jokes about the state and started telling people how wonderful Iowa is.

It was dark when we arrived at our hotel in Iowa City. Clyde checked us into the hotel, finding an entrance close to our first-floor rooms. I was tired from the trip and quickly found a comfortable place to rest in our hotel room recliner. I quickly fell asleep while everyone else visited a restaurant for dinner. I was enjoying my TPN, which I had pumping into my veins twenty-four hours a day. There was no taste, but it kept me alive for more than seven years!

In the morning, we joined the Thompsons for a wonderful continental breakfast in the hotel lobby. The hotel sat right on the banks of the river, with large windows overlooking the river. Bald eagles flew everywhere, nestling in the trees alongside the river. DeeDee loved watching bald eagles glide through the air effortlessly, soaring high in the sky with only a few strokes of their wings. We enjoyed watching the eagles as everyone but me ate breakfast.

The hotel had a shuttle bus to take us to the university. We arrived at the Pappajohn Clinic for my 9:00 a.m. appointment on Monday morning. I know what you are thinking... No, the clinic was not named after the pizza chain restaurant, Papa John's.

Clyde and Karen joined us for the day spent at the clinic. It was very nice for DeeDee to have others with her while they were running tests, ultrasounds, and screening my blood and stomach.

The doctor's nurse was a very special and efficient nurse. After taking my vitals, asking DeeDee and I a hundred or more questions, and reviewing my medical records sent to them by the U of M, I was seen by Dr. Rao.

The first thing he said to us was, "I did not realize you were this sick! We have to do something about this for you." In this examination, he would be inserting a camera and sensor into my stomach. He would review the results tomorrow morning when I returned to his office for more tests.

After inserting the camera and sensor into my stomach, he instructed me to return to the office at 9:00 a.m. the next day. It was a big day; the appointment lasted until 3:00 p.m.! I was very tired and worn out, so I stayed and napped while everyone else went to get something to eat.

I woke up upon their return from the restaurant, visiting with my wife until she fell asleep, and I was awake for the rest of the night! At 9:00 p.m., Dr. Rao called our hotel room and asked if he could stop by my room to make sure the camera and sensor were recording. We planned to meet him in the lobby of the hotel. After ten minutes, he arrived and checked the device on my hip. The camera and sensor were turned off!

Dr. Rao was at his home when he started to ask himself if he had turned the camera on. He was unsettled and decided to check if it was recording, so he drove to the hotel to make sure we would have results for the appointment in the morning. I am glad that God prompted him to do so by the Holy Spirit! Once again, this was a reminder that Jesus had everything under control and that He was looking out for me.

The next day, Dr. Rao removed the camera and sensor from my stomach to review the results. He then asked me to take a breath test, so I was sent to a waiting room with three other men and one woman, who were also taking this test.

We had to breathe into a plastic bag for two minutes and then give the bag to a nurse, who would record the results and levels for Dr. Rao. This was repeated every thirty minutes for four hours. We got to know everyone in the room very well, and we compared our medical stories and complications with each other. I had no idea that so many people faced the same issue as I did with my stomach. After completing the breath test, we were told to return the next day at 9:00 a.m. for a follow-up visit with Dr. Rao.

The next day, we saw Dr. Rao and his nurse for the results. Dr. Rao explained to us, after reviewing all of the tests, that this medical trip to Iowa was an answer from God Almighty to solving a big problem!

With some very positive results from Dr. Rao, we returned to the hotel and checked out of our rooms. Clyde and Karen packed up the motorhome, and we began our trip back to Minnesota.

On the return trip home, I got as comfortable as possible and quickly fell asleep. I think DeeDee, Karen, and Clyde had a big party while I was asleep. I would wake up on occasion to hear laughter and stories. I would drift back asleep, not knowing if they were laughing at me, some good jokes, or an old funny story from the church!

When we arrived back in Northfield, Clyde and Karen helped DeeDee unload all of our gear and luggage from the motorhome, and we thanked them for their time and investment into our lives. The trip would not have been possible without their help!

This was a blessing because DeeDee and I were living on a shoestring budget. I had not received a paycheck in more than five years and was unable to collect Social Security Disability Insurance (SSDI). I had cashed in my retirement and 401(k), using the money to pay bills, but the medical expenses were climbing out of control. DeeDee continued working at the credit union for health insurance coverage, but she transitioned from full-time to part-time to help me with the twenty-four-hour health care I needed.

Clyde and Karen paid for our hotel, the meals at restaurants, and the gasoline for the motorhome. Without their help physically and spiritually on the trip, it would have been very difficult for us. Financially, they were a lifesaver to us, as we were drowning in a debt of medical expenses not paid by the insurance company and the co-pays needed for prescribed drugs. God used them to bless us big time!

I was a terminally ill patient, with no cure for the many medical health problems I had in my body. I was very sick, and I was going downhill every day. God was our only hope (and His people)!

Thank you, Clyde, Karen, Loren, and Shelly Thompson, for your help with this much-needed medical trip. I will never forget your kindness and blessings given to our family. We rejoice together in God's greatness and blessings!

CHAPTER 15
SEVEN YEARS ON A ROLLER COASTER

"The Lord is not slow in keeping his promise, as some understand slowness."
(2 Peter 3:9 NIV)

So far on this health journey, DeeDee and I have experienced between fifty and sixty different hospital stays, most of which were from five to seven days long. Some of them lasted anywhere between fourteen and forty-seven days! It was as if we were riding a roller coaster (something I know a lot about since I built and maintained them many years ago). Our lives have had so many mountaintop experiences and deep, dark valleys with my health.

With monthly infections that started in my stomach and moved into my bloodstream, my body would try to fight them, but my white blood cells could not multiply fast enough. My organs would start shutting down (making me septic), and IV antibiotics had to be given, along with close monitoring of my vitals.

After our appointment with Dr. Rao, the infections got

much better; however, I still had excruciating pain in my mid and right side of my abdomen. The doctors were concerned that it was pancreatitis, which was the reason for the removal of the first pancreas transplant. My pain was still present and very difficult to handle, even with pain medication. I visited my transplant surgeons to consult with them about my abdominal pain, but none of them could decide what to do for me.

I was recommended to see a critical care surgeon named Dr. Beilman. After Dr. Beilman examined me and took MRIs, x-rays, and ultrasounds of my abdomen, he thought it would be a good idea to remove both my appendix and gallbladder. These are not necessary for life, and he wanted them out since they could be the problem.

I was not healthy enough to withstand the two surgeries required to remove the organs, and Dr. Beilman was apprehensive about performing them. After weeks of reviewing my medical records, he decided he would perform the first surgery to remove my appendix.

The same procedures were followed as with my transplant surgeries, with the exception of the length of time involved. Both of the surgeries with Dr. Beilman took only one or two hours. I stayed on the transplant floor for follow-up and care after the surgeries. Dr. Beilman waited until I recovered before removing my gallbladder and the stomach tube and drain in a second surgery.

Dr. Beilman became our hero. He is a very good surgeon with a great bedside manner. He is a very good communicator, careful to weigh all of the options before surgery is performed.

During one of our many hospital stays, I started coughing up clots of blood—some the size of a quarter. My doctor recommended that I see Dr. Hassan, a G.I. specialist at the U of M. After examining me in my hospital room, he believed I had esophageal varices and decided to perform surgery on my esophagus. He used an endoscope to inspect my esophagus and found several varices, which he surgically banded. I was awake and watching everything on the monitor in the procedure room.

After the surgery was completed, I had a sore throat for a day or two. The doctors studied my stomach to rule things out, and they gave me a test to check my motility. The test included me eating an egg traced with radioactive material. They would x-ray my stomach every thirty minutes for two or three hours to see how far the egg had moved through my stomach and intestines.

This test was completed, and the egg did not move through at all. Ten days later, I was in for an x-ray for another health problem when they saw the egg still sitting in my stomach. It had not moved at all. This is when they recommend the stomach tube.

It was decided that I should have a stomach tube installed in my upper abdomen to help with my nutritional needs. When I would eat anything, I would get very ill and throw up, even hours later. They also decided on a drainage tube out of my stomach to collect anything that did not pass through. This would be another minor surgery to install both at the same time, which developed into a major surgery due to my declining health.

The stomach tube and drain were not working. Anything that went into my stomach came right back out of the drainage tube. On Thanksgiving, after eating two spoons of mashed potatoes, DeeDee told me to leave the table and clean up my shirt. The mashed potatoes had flowed right back out and leaked onto my shirt.

I would use one roll of paper towels per day. Every time I

would drink anything, it would flow out of the tube and the bag meant to catch it, leaking onto my clothes. I would take four pieces of paper towels, fold them in half and then quarter them, and stick the towels into the waistband of the pants I was wearing to catch the fluids flowing out of my stomach. I was getting no nutrition in my body from food or drink. It was decided that I go on TPN only, and they removed my feeding tube.

I did not eat anything for over a five-year period of time. Nothing went into my mouth to eat. Watching television was difficult because about half of the commercials were food- or restaurant-related. The food products looked so good on the television ads!

Following this, I came down with very painful, burning sores on the left side of my body, from my chest down to my knee. This was a very intense burning sensation and left open sores, which broke open and drained. It was diagnosed as shingles. If you had the mumps as a child, the shingle virus lives in your body. When your immune system weakens, the virus grows into a shingles attack.

I had severe nerve pain from this virus for more than two years. Remember that my immune system was medicated to stop the white blood cells from attacking the donor pancreas graft? My immune system never recovered after two years of taking CellCept.

The lymphedema in my lower legs was closely watched. The fluid in my lower legs expanded, and the skin on my lower legs turned black and blue from poor circulation. I was prescribed many different creams and ointments to apply to my skin. Our daughter, Alanna, recommended that we use coconut oil, which really helped! Our wound care nurse couldn't believe the difference in the condition of my skin and sores after several weeks of its use.

With these drug interactions, I was assigned a sitter in my

room from the hospital. They did not want me to harm myself. Please keep in mind that I did not leave my bed— they were concerned for my mind. DeeDee watched me closely and judged whether I was in my right mind or not. You need someone to advocate for you when you cannot speak for yourself. You need help when you are overmedicated, undermedicated, or experiencing unusual behavior from a drug interaction.

DeeDee watched over my mental and physical health needs. She could tell what was going on with me because she knew me better than anyone else. If I was sleeping too long during the day, she would inform the doctors that I was overmedicated. Once they changed the dosage, I would stop sleeping twenty hours a day. If a drug made my mind kind of loopy—if I was talking crazy and not making sense—she would tell the doctors, and they would choose another drug. Many times, these drugs have side effects, some minor and others extreme.

Everyone needs somebody to be an advocate for them. Someone has to ask the tough questions and help with the physical, emotional, or spiritual needs of life. DeeDee and I, along our journey, have spent every holiday celebration in the hospital. It was not all in the same year, but every holiday, birthday, anniversary, birth, and death took place while I was in the hospital.

When my mother was moved from her home into an end-of-life facility two days before she died, I requested to be discharged from the hospital so I could be with her. The doctors and hospital approved, although I was very ill at the time. Everyone knew my mother and loved her.

When I arrived home that afternoon of November 10, 2010, we drove to the facility to visit Mother. She was so happy to see me—she could not believe that I was there with her. She knew I was hospitalized because DeeDee had visited with her at the house a few days before. When Mom saw me in the room, she said, "Am I seeing things, or are you really here?"

As we visited, I told Mom how much she meant to us, how much we loved her, and how we appreciated her love and care for me. When my mother was diagnosed with ovarian cancer, we had talked about which one of us would beat the other one to Heaven and meet Jesus first. My mother looked into my eyes that evening before her death and said, "I am going to beat you!"

A little after noon on November 11, 2010, my dad, my brother, Tom, and I were sitting with Mom in the hospice room when she breathed her last breath on this earth, quietly slipping from this life into eternal life with Christ Jesus, our Lord and Savior.

DeeDee and Alanna had gone to the grocery store to pick up food for everyone. They prepared lunch for the family members who had gathered together with Mom. We had been at the facility since early in the morning. DeeDee was serving everyone in a dining room down the hall from Mom's room when she died.

Mom would have done the same thing as DeeDee and Alanna—serving and taking care of people's needs were always on her mind. Mom would always make and serve food for others. Mother left this earth only when she knew that DeeDee and Alanna had served lunch for her family.

God gave me strength to make the funeral arrangements and to officiate her funeral service at church. We had discussed our funeral arrangements with each other before she died, so I performed the service as per her wishes. After the service, I was readmitted to the hospital for care.

The social workers and medical staff began to recommend to DeeDee that I go into hospice care or be placed in a transitional facility. The hospital did not expect me to live. I, on the other hand, wanted only to be home and trust God for my healing.

For more than a year, I was taking fentanyl lollipops for pain along with oral dilaudid for pain. The lollipops were only for terminally ill cancer patients, but they made an exception for me because of the constant abdominal pain. The lollipops were in my mouth twenty-four hours a day! However, the side effect was that they destroyed my teeth.

Over this seven-year period of time, I was in a wheelchair for more than a year, a walker for two years, and used an IV pole as a cane for five years. I am very thankful for the way God has restored my ability to walk without assistance after more than seven years of needing this help.

Now, when doctors look into my medical charts or access them on the computer, it takes nearly ten minutes to show up on the computer screen. I have over five thousand pages of medical records. The doctors enter my account on the computer, go on a coffee break, and return ten minutes later to view my records. When I go in for any surgery, five thousand pages of medical records are loaded onto my bed, joining me in the operating room.

This rollercoaster ride was not cheap; you would not believe the medical costs of my health care! The cost of medical treatments for terminally ill patients has exploded, and it looks like it's only going higher with no drop in sight.

The cost of my prescription drugs (for my oral pills only) was over nine thousand dollars a month. To add in the weekly injections of Aranesp to raise my hemoglobin, it was another five or six thousand dollars per month. The TPN and supplies were over ten thousand dollars a month. When you add it all up, the total cost of medications was over twenty-five thousand dollars per month, or three hundred thousand dollars per year!

To live with major health issues in your body, you need

very good health insurance! DeeDee stayed working for this reason. Over my journey, our health insurance company paid out over six million dollars for my care. That's why I refer to myself as the "Six-Million-Dollar Man!" The Lord was the only one I saw that could get me off this rollercoaster and back on solid ground.

CHAPTER 16
FATHER'S DAY OF 2014

"Be joyful in hope, patient in affliction, faithful in prayer."
(Romans 12:12 NIV)

The week after Memorial Day was June 2, 2014. I was mowing the lawn at our home, riding our John Deere lawn mower. We do not have a large lawn, but I was not able to walk behind a push mower. Over the years, my legs became very weak. Mowing the lawn wore me out for the day, even when using the riding mower!

I was wearing shorts that day. I did not feel it, but a few tiny mosquitoes had bitten me on my left knee. My body over the last year began reacting badly to mosquito bites. The bites would swell up very large, to the size of a dime, and they would itch like crazy!

Five or seven days later, my left knee became infected from these bites. I had been using every drug available in our home pharmacy to stop the itching, but nothing seemed to work.

It was six days before Father's Day. In the early morning

hours of June 9, I woke DeeDee up at 1:00 a.m., asking her to take my temperature because I was burning up. My temperature was one hundred and one degrees. I was nauseous and throwing up, and I could not keep down my oral pain medication. I asked DeeDee to take me to the hospital because I knew I had a bad infection in my body. We arrived at the ER at 3:00 a.m.

When they weighed me and took my vitals at the check-in desk, I weighed one hundred and ninety pounds. I was very frustrated with my weight over the last seven years—I normally weighed one hundred and thirty-five pounds, but I was retaining so much fluid from the TPN, had not eaten anything in seven years, and could do nothing about the fluid buildup. Even with diuretics, I kept retaining fluids.

After I was brought into an examination room, I was given IV pain medication with the dosage prescribed on the doctor's letter we gave to the ER doctor. I was so sick; I laid in bed and fell asleep.

DeeDee was my advocate. She made sure I had a private room on the medicine floor because the transplant floor was full. I was assigned a new doctor, Dr. Song.

The nurses were wonderful, and the doctors were concerned. The lab techs drew my blood, running tests for the type of infection I had. In the meantime, my organs began to shut down—I was septic. I laid in bed from Monday morning to Sunday afternoon.

When Dr. Song and his crew of medical students and doctors (fellows and interns) examined me on Tuesday morning, they discussed my septic condition. DeeDee asked him if she could go to work tomorrow, which was about thirty minutes away. Dr. Song replied, "I would prefer that you not go to work tomorrow. I do not think you will have enough time to get back here to say goodbye to your husband!"

Dr. Song and the other doctors did not expect me to live. After the medical students, interns, pharmacist, and Dr. Song left the room, DeeDee made a call to the charge nurse on the transplant floor. A private room was available for me, so transport moved me in my bed to the transplant floor, where all of the nurses and staff knew DeeDee and I very well.

After being moved to my room, I was well taken care of by the nurses we loved and knew so well. They did everything they could to make me comfortable and also cared for DeeDee. The nurses were her support group and had become her friends.

I was having a very difficult time breathing, and the oxygen level was turned up as high as it would go in my room. My heart was very erratic. Technicians took x-rays of my chest and lungs while I lay in bed. The heart technicians took several EKGs during the day to run comparisons on how my heart was functioning.

My kidneys had already shut down. I had not urinated since giving a urine sample for a test in the ER at 3:00 a.m. on Monday morning. I was retaining fluid. Even though the nurses were giving me diuretics to remove the fluid, my kidneys were not working.

DeeDee had to communicate for me. I was so ill that all I could do was lay in the hospital bed, pray, and quote scriptures to myself. DeeDee had notified everyone to pray for me. So many faithful friends prayed and sent messages to us!

When Dr. Song and the crew visited my room on Wednesday morning, they were a little surprised that I was still hanging on to life. The doctor had started me on vancomycin, which is a heavy-duty antibiotic used to get my many infections under control. The doctors were watching my heart and my lungs, along with the output from my kidneys.

On Wednesday evening at 8:00 p.m., my nurse for the evening was a man. I had only seen him once or twice before. He came into my room to hang a new bag of TPN for me, hooking up one of the lines into my PICC line. He had to leave my room to get some more supplies to attach the lipids to the other port in my PICC line.

When he left the room, DeeDee was working on her computer. It was then that I heard the voice from Heaven. Honestly, I do not know if the voice was God or His son, Jesus. I had heard this same voice before when God called us into the ministry.

This audible voice was the same one we had both heard before. DeeDee had heard it when she disconnected me from my life support machines. This voice is unmistakable! When God speaks to you in an audible voice, please listen and be obedient to what He is telling you!

This is what I heard the Lord say: "Do not let them give you any IV fluids, or you will die!" I turned my head to DeeDee to ask her if she heard that. "Hear what?" she asked me. I responded, "Nevermind, I know who was talking to me!"

We have never been afraid to die—to be absent from the body is to be present with the Lord (2 Corinthians 5:8). I love spending time with my children and grandchildren. I also enjoy time with my beautiful, wonderful wife. But I do know this: *when God Himself speaks to me in an audible voice, I should listen and obey the words spoken to me!*

When the nurse returned to my hospital room, I told him, "There is no need for you to hook up the lipids. I refuse all IV fluids! Please disconnect my lines flowing into the ports of my PICC line." The nurse thought I was giving up on life after ten years! He thought I was ending my life with a dignified suicide. They knew that I received all of my nutrition through my veins. Without TPN, I would not live long. The nurse wrote in my chart, "Patient refuses all IV fluids!"

I asked the nurse to bring a scale into my room to weigh me, which was something I never wanted to do. When I was weighed in the clinic or doctor's office, I would not look at the scale and ask the nurse not to tell me my weight.

I knew I was retaining fluids. My wrist, fingers, arms, legs, and chest were very large and swollen. When I stepped out of bed for the first time in days, I got on the scale and was shocked at my weight: two hundred and sixteen pounds. I had gained twenty-six pounds of fluid in three days—no wonder why my heart and lungs were working so hard. All of the fluid on my chest was making it very difficult for my heart and lungs, so they were working overtime!

Death by crucifixion was a very painful process. Most people actually died from asphyxiation, the weight of their bodies pushing on the lungs. People nailed or tied to a cross would try to push up with their legs to relieve the pressure on their lungs and to simply get one good breath of air. I could feel what it must have been like for them.

For three days—Thursday, Friday, and Saturday—I simply laid in bed and slept as the nurses and doctors treated me. DeeDee did go to work on Friday. I was still very ill, and my kidneys were not working. I was not able to remove the fluids from my body through urination.

While I was in the hospital, I developed a blood clot on the end of my PICC line, near my heart. If the blood clot broke loose, it would flow to my heart or lungs, and I would die.

The line needed to be removed. I had kept this PICC line in my arm for two years, which was a record number of days (they usually are not in for more than two or three months). I had run out of veins to use—this was my last vein! They do not tell you that you can run out of veins for PICC lines. I was terminally ill and was not expected to live long enough to run out of veins.

Without a PICC line, I could not have TPN, and I needed both to survive! They can put a line in your neck, which I had with many of my surgeries, but it is not used for any extended length of time because it easily gets infected.

The doctors were still very concerned with my septic condition. Many times, I could only open my eyes when they examined me or checked my pupils for dilation responses. DeeDee had to speak for me. For four days, I did not have any IV fluids.

Sunday, June 15, was Father's Day! I had been in the hospital for six days, laying in the hospital bed and sleeping most of the time. Our daughter, Alanna, called after church and spoke with DeeDee. Alanna and her family wanted to stop by the hospital to see me. The grandchildren—Gavin, Grady, Gracyn, and Georgia Grace —were missing PaPa and MeMaw. After all, it was Father's Day!

DeeDee asked me if they could visit, and I said yes. We asked them to call us when they arrived at valet parking. I always tried to appear the best I could with our seven grand-children. I did not want them to remember me as always being sick, laying in bed, and dying.

I fell asleep in bed, and an hour or so later, we received the telephone call that they were at valet parking. I asked DeeDee to help me get out of bed and walk me into the bathroom, where I washed my face and brushed my teeth. I was standing by the side of the bed when everyone walked into the hospital room.

I was disconnected from the oxygen and all of the fluids, which they were used to seeing me with. I played with them, visited with them, and enjoyed looking at the cards and pictures they had drawn for me. It was a great Father's Day!

Our oldest daughter, Shanna, and our grandchildren, Blake Madison, Noah, and CJ, called me an hour or so later.

I was worn out! I had not gotten out of bed but once before during the six days in the hospital. I was so tired from standing up and playing with the kids. I felt better physically, but I was very tired. I asked DeeDee to help me get back into bed. When I laid back down, I quickly fell asleep.

After an hour or two, I felt a sensation in my body, which I had not felt in six or seven days. I asked DeeDee to help me get up to the bathroom. When I got there, I knew I had to use the urinal because they measure everything in the hospital! God bless the nurses and medical staff who have to measure and check everything that goes in and out of your body. I filled one urinal and had to ask for another one to fill.

When my nurse came into the room a short time later, she asked us where all of the urine came from. When DeeDee told her, our nurse was very surprised. I had gone from producing nothing to overfilling the containers. My kidneys started working, and I was feeling great by late evening.

I fell asleep that afternoon and slept through the night. On Monday morning, I woke up with DeeDee at 5:00 a.m., got out of bed, got dressed, and kissed her goodbye. When she left for work, I told her she could take me home when she arrived back at the hospital.

When Dr. Song and the crew arrived in my hospital room, they were shocked! I was standing up by the bed—he had only seen me laying in the bed for the last seven days. I told him that I wanted my discharge papers signed before DeeDee picked me up at 4:30 p.m. Dr. Song replied, "I can't let you go home. You are here with us for another five-seven days!" I told him that I had gone home much sicker than this. After examining me and starting a round of oral antibiotics, Dr. Song said that he would check my blood tests, review my charts from the weekend, and get back with me.

My nurse was Andrea, whom we had known for years. She started out as an aid, attended nursing school at the U of M, and became a great registered nurse. I told her to keep an eye out for my discharge orders from Dr. Song on the computer. She took great care of me!

When DeeDee arrived after work, I had everything packed up and was ready to leave. We continued to check the computer for an update about my discharge papers.

At 7:00 p.m., I started walking the halls, looking for a doctor, when I heard Dr. Song's voice in an office, talking on the telephone with his wife. I knocked on the door, opened it, and walked in. "I need my discharge orders, Dr. Song!" I said. He looked at me and said, "I can't let you go home." I told him that he would need to talk to DeeDee. He told me to send her down to see him.

DeeDee walked down to his office, where Dr. Song told her the same thing. She reasoned with him that I had gone home sicker than this and in worse condition, assuring him that if I got worse, she would bring me back to the hospital. "We do not want him to catch something in the hospital and stay longer," she explained. "Carl will do better at home. He will rest better, and I will take care of him like the nurses do."

To this, Dr. Song said, "If it were anyone else, I would not let Carl go home. I know you have taken good care of him for ten years. Promise me that if he gets worse, you will bring him back to the hospital." We left the hospital at 9:00 p.m. that evening.

On the drive home in the car, I told DeeDee, "I am not taking anymore TPN. I do not want any IV fluids." When we arrived home, I took a big breath of air. It felt so good to walk into our home and climb into our own bed. I was so hungry after being without food or nutrition since Wednesday, when they disconnected me from all IV fluids. I ate yogurt before I went to bed, and it tasted so good! I closed my eyes, thanking

God for His words spoken to me in the hospital room. I prayed myself to sleep that night.

Please note: *I do not recommend anyone stop taking their medications! Please consult with your physician before stopping any medications in your life. I consulted with my doctor, and he advised me to continue with the twice-a-week blood draws and tests. I assured him that I would restart TPN if my lab results were not improving.*

CHAPTER 17
OFF TPN COLD TURKEY

"Dear friend, I pray that you may enjoy good health and that all may go well with you, even as your soul is getting along well."
(3 John 2 NIV)

It was early in the morning of Tuesday, June 17, 2014, when I quit everything cold turkey. I stopped taking all my medications. I had been without TPN since Wednesday night, making six nights without nutrition for my body. I started eating yogurt and clear soups, giving my digestive system a restart.

I stopped my oral pain medications, which I had taken for over ten years, every two hours. The pain clinic told me that they reduce your dosage very slowly for a month at a time, let your body reset its pain tolerance for a month, and then continue until you are off of your medications. This process would have taken me almost three years.

I started drinking a high-protein shake each day. Derek and Alanna, along with our grandchildren, had been drinking them for seven years.

My home care nurse, Alison, drew my labs on Tuesday,

and I was shocked with the results. My numbers looked better than ever. Alison was happy to see me home again. She didn't know I was off TPN at this point.

The next day, I had a follow-up doctor's appointment with Dr. Sick. When he saw me, he said that I looked different from the other follow-ups and hospitalizations. I showed him my labs and explained that I hadn't had TPN for a week. He shook his head in disbelief. I told Dr. Sick that I would not take IV fluids anymore.

He looked at DeeDee and me, responding, "Alright. Keep this between us only. Do not tell anyone what we are doing. We will try a trial or an experiment. Continue with your twice-a-week blood draws and tests. If the numbers start going down, you will need to start TPN again. Do not let the home infusion people know you are not taking TPN. Let them continue to mix your TPN based on your current blood draws. You will need to use the new TPN mix, if needed."

Dr. Sick told us that he was going on a two-week vacation and then speaking at a convention for a week. He planned to see me as soon as he got back into town. If my numbers went down during this time, I agreed to use TPN again.

When we left his office, we stopped at the front desk for a follow-up appointment. Dr. Sick was very busy and was currently not taking on any new patients in his practice. The earliest appointment we could get was six weeks away. We took the appointment and left for home.

I was feeling stronger each day and slowly losing the fluid weight from the hospital stay. I was working on my bending and stretching. I was walking and doing a few more things around the house. Each day, I became healthier and better.

I have to thank our grandson, Grady, who was playing with some Hot Wheels on the floor in our living room one day. He looked at me and said, "PaPa, I want you to get down on the floor and play with me!" I looked at Grady and said, "I would love to, honey, but if I got down on the floor, I would not be able to stand back up again! I can't bend at the waist anymore."

Grady looked me in the eyes. "Poppy, you have to have a goal. You have to start somewhere!" Grady's gentle words cut me like a knife. He was right; I had to start bending at the waist in order to break up the scar tissue.

I started bending at the waist and touching my knees. It was a start, like Grady had said. I also set some goals for myself: to go swimming with Gavin and Grady at the end of summer and to be able to put on my own socks and shoes by myself.

It was a work in progress, and I loved each and every day because I was able to do more things than in the past ten years.

All of our grandchildren were so good for me, encouraging me through this whole process. I always enjoyed their company, no matter how tired or worn out I was. I would rise up to meet them and have fun with them. I loved spending time with each one of them, whether playing games or simply watching them play.

DeeDee and I kept our secret experiment to ourselves, and we continued to rejoice as I got better and better. I had some bad days when I overdid something, but life was good!

On Sunday, July 27, 2014, I was able to put on a pair of socks and shoes by myself for the first time in over ten years. It took me ten or fifteen minutes, but I was able to do this simple task without help from anyone else.

I know many people put their socks and shoes on without even thinking about it. They can do it with their eyes closed. For men like me, it is very difficult to ask for help with such a simple task, but the truth is, we all need help from time to time. I know our help comes from the Lord, but He sent wonderful people to help, like my wife, my nurse, and even my grandkids. I realized the Lord was using them to help and bless me. So many times, we want a pill or a quick fix when God is using a process. Yes, it was a slow process at times, but God was not only healing me; He was teaching me how to be thankful for even the little things. He is the one who leads us in steps!

Dr. Brian Sick has been a continuous blessing to DeeDee and me. He coordinated my healthcare, working with my twelve specialists to decide on treatments that would be helpful to me. He has been a lifesaver and a great decision-maker for us.

While Dr. Sick was away for three weeks, I continued with my blood draws and tests. I monitored the results very closely as the fax machine printed off the results of my blood tests biweekly. I impatiently waited for the page to finish printing so I could turn the page over and rejoice with the test results.

With each blood test, my numbers improved. They were not going down; they were on a steady increase to much improved health. It was fun to see the numbers now in the normal range.

DeeDee and I felt a little strange not telling my home care nurse, Alison, why my numbers were improving. She was in shock at the drastic improvement in each blood draw.

When I would speak to our home infusion pharmacist, Lori, I felt as though I was deceiving her. She was excited about the improved numbers in my blood tests. I felt awkward explaining to Lori how I was improving in health or why we saw such drastic improvement in the blood tests.

I felt bad when Lori mixed up the new TPN recipe for my blood draws. When the courier dropped the TPN off at our home, I drained the old recipe of TPN down into the sink. I was following the doctor's orders!

It had now been six weeks since I had seen Dr. Sick, and it

was time for my appointment. I had not had any IV fluids for seven weeks. I brought my lab results taken the day before with me. When Dr. Sick walked into the examination room and saw me, he was taken completely by surprise!

He looked at me and said, "I cannot believe how good you look! In seven years, I have never seen you look this good!" I shook Dr. Sick's hand as he sat down in his chair next to me before handing him the lab results.

As he reviewed the numbers, he could not believe it! He looked at me with a shocked look in his eyes and a huge smile on his face. "I cannot believe this! These numbers are unbelievable—I guess our little trial was successful!" I looked at him and told him, "God healed me!"

Dr. Sick knew that DeeDee and I were believers. He knew that we were very positive in our attitudes, even when we received negative news. He examined me, checked my vitals, and shook his head in disbelief. "I cannot believe this. I have no medical explanation for the healing. It must be God!"

He went to his desk and began typing on his keyboard to update my medical chart. He sent a message to Fairview Home Infusion: "Trial successful! Discontinue TPN. Patient is now eating for nutrition."

A memo was also sent to the radiologists: "Please remove the PICC line as soon as possible. Carl wants to go swimming and jump into the lake with his grandchildren!" An appointment was scheduled for August 8 to remove the line. I had a PICC line in one of my arms for over ten years. I couldn't wait to have it removed!

Dr. Sick thanked DeeDee for all of her wonderful care for me over the years. I asked him when he'd like to see me again, to which he said three months. We also were to stop the twice-a-week blood draws, transitioning to just once a month.

I could not believe it. I had blood tests twice a week

during this whole ordeal. Now I was giving blood only once a month!

Upon our arrival back at the house, the telephone rang. DeeDee answered the telephone, and I heard the voice of Lori, the pharmacist, on the other end of the line. Lori was crying because she was so excited about the news from the doctor.

Lori explained that I held the record—I was the only one who had been on TPN for more than seven years. Most people are on TPN for a month or two. Usually, people die after one or two years of this treatment. It is not normal to receive your nutrition through your veins.

She told DeeDee that they would not know what to do on Mondays or Thursdays now that they did not have to mix my TPN. Everyone at Fairview Home Infusion would ask each other on Mondays and Thursdays, "Has anyone seen Carl's labs yet?" They looked forward to mixing my TPN and getting it out to me twice a week.

It was an experience that I will never forget. Our children and grandchildren wondered if this was for real or not. We experienced so many mountaintop joys and many deep, dark valleys over the years. With many of these health problems, we simply took a "wait and see" attitude! We believed in God as our healer.

Over the next two weeks until my radiologist appointment, we all patiently waited for the last step in my healing! The removal of the PICC line from my body was the last device still in my body.

I continued to grow stronger and healthier each and every day. However, I was careful not to overdo things because I would pay for it later. My creatinine numbers for my kidneys were now near normal. From stage-four kidney disease to near-normal levels within a tenth of a point above normal was a miracle from God Almighty.

DeeDee and I rejoiced with each month's blood tests. What a joy it was for us to see God at work in my life. We serve a God of restoration and healing through the sacrifice of Christ Jesus, our Lord and Savior. Jesus paid the penalty for our sins and for our healing on the Cross of Calvary. To God be the glory!

CHAPTER 18
MY HAIRCUT AND CELEBRATION

"Rejoice in the Lord always. I will say it again: Rejoice!"
(Philippians 4:4 NIV)

Exactly two years to the date when the radiologist installed my PICC line in my left arm, they removed it! I went into the procedure room where they hooked up all of the monitors and prepared me for the next steps. I laid down on the table with my arm draped and ready for the removal, waiting for the radiologist to arrive in the procedure room.

I had a blood clot at the end of my PICC line, which they had to double check before pulling it. They did not want the clot to break loose and enter my heart or lungs. They injected dye into my line, checking it with their equipment. After checking, the doctor told me that he could not see any blood clots present. God had removed the blood clot for me!

The doctor simply pulled the PICC line out, wiped the site with an alcohol wipe, and put a bandage on top. Everyone congratulated me. This was the first time in over ten years that I left the procedure room without a PICC line in my body.

As I walked out of the hospital that day, I walked out of the door with only what God had given me in my body when I was born. I had no other devices or any foreign objects in my body—it felt so good! I met DeeDee, and we celebrated!

Our grandchildren were so encouraging and brought me so much happiness over the years. We wanted to celebrate the healing miracle of God Almighty with them and our children, Shanna and Alanna.

DeeDee called our friend, Pam Heikkila, who was also our family photographer, to see if we could stop by her studio and shoot some photos. I had made a vow to God about five years prior that I would not cut my hair until I was healed. This way, when people saw me with short hair, they would know automatically that God had healed me.

This was finally the day to celebrate and cut my hair, and I wanted our grandchildren to do the honors!

We arrived at Heikkila Photography Studio and quickly began the celebration with all seven of our grandchildren. They sprayed bright-colored hair spray on their white shirts. After spraying me down with color, we were ready for the spiked hair!

Our oldest granddaughter, Blake Madison, cut my ponytail off as the others watched and cheered! The ponytail was three feet long! My hair was so long that it was past my waist.

We had a lot of fun celebrating the wonderful gift of healing. After the photo session, we went out to eat, further celebrating the miracle from God, our healer (Psalm 30:2)!

DeeDee and I then went home so I could prepare for Sunday morning. We were to give the testimony of God's healing in my life at our home church's morning service.

During the service, DeeDee and I shared how God healed

me many times over the past ten-plus years. We declared that God "is the same yesterday, today, and forever." God does not change. God still heals us and helps us when we pray!

With God, all things are possible. Nothing is too difficult for God. When we put our faith in Him, He helps us in our times of trouble. We can ask anything in His name, and it shall be done—according to His will!

After our testimony of God's healing power in my life, we asked for people who wanted prayer to come forward to the altar area of the church. I looked at the clock and it was 11:45 a.m.

We called for the elders and pastors of the church to join us as we prayed for people's needs. We anointed them with oil, as James 5 instructs us, and we prayed for physical, emotional, and spiritual needs.

As we finished praying for the people's needs, I looked at the clock—the time was 1:00 p.m. We prayed at the altar with people for seventy-five minutes. This does not happen in today's churches!

Some people in the church had left, but the majority of the people stayed and prayed under the sweet spirit of the Lord Jesus. His presence was very strong in the church, and the anointing of the Holy Spirit freely flowed, helping people with their needs.

God met with us and met many of the needs of His people. Russ Hatten was the last person I prayed with that Sunday morning. Two weeks later, Russ told me what God had done for him.

He had come up to the altar for prayer, and I asked him what he wanted prayer for. Russ explained that after moving into his new condominium, he had to climb up five stairs to enter through the front door. Each time he walked up the steps, he experienced several seconds of chest pain. He had seen his cardiologist, Dr. Panetta (we shared the same doctor), who tested his heart, but it turned out that the heart was not the problem.

Russ saw a neurologist, who found a leak in a vein near his brain. Each time Russ walked up the stairs, his heart pumped harder to send blood to the brain through a vein that was leaking out the blood.

The doctor told Russ that he would not die from this leak, but it was too close to the motor skills of his brain. They did not recommend surgery because of the danger of losing motor skill functions, like his ability to walk or talk.

After praying and releasing our faith together, we believed God for His healing hand to touch and heal Russ' body and leaky vein. When Russ arrived home, he went up the stairs and did not have any chest pain. He continued going up and down the stairs for two weeks. After that time, Russ told me how God had healed his body.

At first, he was afraid to tell me for fear he would "jinks" himself. I told Russ, "When God heals you, you are healed!"

Another lady in our church had severe stomach problems and had gone to two different doctors, both of whom could not help her. She came up for prayer, and she went home healed! She struggled to keep anything down in her stomach, except for yogurt and clear liquids, but she started eating. By Wednesday morning, she was eating normal food again after months of problems.

God healed her, like Russ, miraculously! Jesus paid for their healing on the Cross of Calvary. By His stripes, we are healed—all for His glory and honor!

Many others were healed in church through the gift of healing. This is a restorative gift from God. When we cut our finger with a knife, God causes the blood to clot to stop the bleeding. He causes the tissue to grow back together after several days, restoring our health. Many times, the gift of healing takes time.

Let me give you an example: building a car on the assembly line. A new car can be built in a matter of minutes. However, to restore a car, it takes weeks, months, and, many times, years to restore it to like-new or better-than-new condition. Rebuilders must disassemble every part of the car, rebuilding each one, before reassembling it.

We have continued to see God heal miraculously when we share this testimony, and we believe God will also restore our state, nation, and world.

The very next day, my home care nurse, Alison Valenski, arrived at our door for our twice-a-week blood draw and tests. When she opened the door and saw me with my haircut, she knew that I was healed!

She could not believe it! Alison looked at my arm, seeing there was no PICC line installed, and asked me, "What am I going to do?" I replied back, "You better call Fairview Home Infusion for your orders." When she called them, they told her that I no longer needed home health care!

She turned to me and said, "I won't know what to do on Monday and Thursday mornings anymore. You were always my first patient. My car will automatically turn down your street and stop at your house. I have been seeing you for more than eight years."

I thanked her, as I always have, telling her what a good job she did and how we would miss her smiling face. I thanked her for all of the difficult health problems she had helped us gain the victory over. I told her how much we appreciated her and her cheerful, wonderful attitude.

It was difficult for both of us to say goodbye. After eight years together, you become friends with each other. Alison said there were times over the eight years when she did not think I would ever come home from the hospital. She was shocked each time I came home with more IV medicine and new drugs to take. She shared with us that our positive attitudes in the worst of situations made all the difference in the world. We finally said goodbye to each other with tears in our eyes and happiness in our hearts!

CHAPTER 19
OUR LIFE TODAY

"By his wounds you have been healed."
(1 Peter 2:24 NIV)

As I am writing this, nine years have passed since God miraculously healed me on Father's Day, June 15, 2014. I have grown stronger and healthier each and every day. I am glad to tell you that my blood tests have improved each month to near-normal and normal levels. I now have my labs drawn every six months. My immune system is much improved, and my creatinine levels are now normal at 1.3!

I was able to complete both of my goals, which our grandson, Grady, helped me with. I was able to put my own socks and shoes on without any assistance from anyone, and I was able to go swimming with our grandsons, Gavin and Grady, in the swimming pool at the YMCA on September 6, 2014. The doctor asked me to please not jump into the lake because of the possible infections from the lake water. I try to follow the doctor's orders!

Gavin, Grady, and I swam together for nearly three hours

in the pool. The boys had never seen me without my bag of TPN fluid attached to one of my arms. We swam in the pool, played water basketball, swam for objects at the bottom of the pool, and went down the water slide. It was the first time I had been in a swimming pool in over fifteen years. Boy, was it fun!

All of our grandkids had to get used to the new PaPa. I was now able to be a normal, healthy grandparent to them. I always tried to be as normal as possible, but now they see me in a new light!

I did need some help to improve my leg muscles. I asked Dr. Sick for a physical therapy consultation, and he gladly gave me the evaluation order. I visited a physical therapist in Northfield named Maria. She worked with me at the swimming pool to strengthen my leg muscles and break down the scar tissue in my abdomen.

After nine weeks of physical therapy, I was like the little engine that could. I kept telling myself, "I think I can! I think I can! I know I can! I know I can!" When Maria measured the divot in my abdomen from the scar, it had all but flattened out after she broke down my scar tissue. I was amazed and felt great!

I started doing more household tasks around the house. I even scraped and painted the house by myself. Climbing the ladder was a little tricky, but I succeeded. The house looked great! I also raked the leaves for the first time in over a decade. I think it was all driving DeeDee a bit crazy since she is still very protective of me! God bless her (and He does)!

My digestive system took a while to kick in. Two days after I started eating again, I was eating cheese pizza—a real treat after all these years of not eating! I am now eating almost everything. I have a little problem with steaks, red meat, rough vegetables, and salads, but some of these are not really good for us anyway.

It was fun for DeeDee after all these years to finally have someone to eat with. It was hard for her to cook for herself. It is not really rewarding to eat by yourself. We enjoy dining together and talking over our meals together.

In November, we celebrated Thanksgiving, Gavin's favorite holiday! I was able to eat this Thanksgiving after years of smelling the wonderful food. I enjoyed turkey with stuffing, mashed potatoes and gravy, sweet potatoes, green bean casserole, cheesy potatoes, cranberry sauce, rolls, and pie for dessert. What a treat! I had to try a spoonful of everything on the table. I was very thankful for God's healing on this Thanksgiving! I am now "Thanks-living" every day, not just one day a year. I continue to live my life daily, thankful to God for His precious gift of life!

I included working out and exercising into my new daily routine to help my muscles and tissues get back in shape. I have lost over eighty pounds since my weigh-in at the hospital on the night God spoke to me. I am now balanced out at one hundred and thirty-five pounds—the same as I weighed a little over ten years ago. I am so glad to store away the extra, extra-large shirts DeeDee and Alanna had bought for me to wear.

People today ask me how I lost weight, to which I tell them, "You do not want to go on the diet I was on for the last decade!" I now realize how hard it is to lose weight. It is one thing to talk about it and another thing to do it. I tried everything I could—I even asked the pharmacist to lower the calories in my TPN bag—but I was simply retaining the fluid because my kidneys were not working properly.

I saw my nephrologist, Dr. Kukla, in mid-January of 2015 in the hallway at the U of M. When she saw me, she said, "Carl Lindelien, what happened to you?" That's when I told her that God had healed me. She looked me in the eyes, asking what my creatinine level was.

Medical staff can check kidney function with a simple blood test. The normal creatinine level in the blood is between 1.1 and 1.5, and mine was always three or four times above normal. I informed Dr. Kukla that my creatinine was 1.3. That is right in the middle of normal, and I have never been normal with anything in my life!

That is when she told me that I no longer had kidney disease. I looked into her eyes and said, "Thank you, doctor. This is what I wanted to hear!" As Dr. Kukla walked away from me, she looked back over her shoulder, wanting to say more, but smiled and kept walking down the hall.

Of all my twelve specialists, I see them only in the hallways of the U of M, and I always say hello to them. They call me the "Miracle Man" there. What a joy it is to walk down a hallway and see the look on their faces when they see DeeDee and me walking together.

Our conversations always begin with the doctors and medical staff. They say, "I cannot believe it. You look so good. I would never have imagined seeing you like this!"

Micah Heikkila, one of my prayer warriors at church, is thirteen years old and has prayed for me every day and night for many years. He asked me a question after God healed me: *Was it worth it?* "Yes!" I told him. "If one person's life is changed, or we can help encourage one person because of the trials we have been through, it is worth everything!" Micah looked into my eyes, smiled, and replied, "I thought you would say something like that."

Today, God has restored me to a full-time ministry position with the Minnesota District Council of the Assemblies of God. We are "U.S. home missionaries" as pastoral care pastors. We have two hundred and fifty-plus churches and over one thousand ministers of the gospel, whom we partner with to help people with their health care and life's problems.

We call on the twenty-two metro hospitals in the Twin

Cities of Minneapolis and St. Paul, nursing and retirement homes, hospice care, state prisons, county jails, home visits, and shut-ins. I enjoy each and every visit sharing God's love, hope, encouragement, faith, and prayer with people who, many times, are desperate for God's help in their times of trouble.

God is blessing and restoring us like our heroes from the Bible. I love believing and praying with people for their needs to be met by Jesus Christ and by the power of the Holy Spirit. Nothing is too hard for God Almighty!

To God be the glory, forever and ever! *Amen and amen.*

"For I am the LORD, who heals you." (Exodus 15:26 NIV)

CHAPTER 20
WHAT TO SAY TO SOMEONE

"May the God of hope fill you with all joy and peace as you trust in him, so that you may overflow with hope by the power of the Holy Spirit."
(Romans 15:13 NIV)

Sometimes it is hard to find the right words to say. Here are some helpful suggestions for what you can say to a patient or their family when you visit them in the hospital or at home!

<u>Within the Hospital</u>:

Be positive in your words and comments. Start the conversation with something like, "It is so good to see you," "You look good," "I am so happy to see you smiling," or "Your eyes look bright!" Don't lie, but find positive things to say to the person!

While I was in the hospital with different surgeries, I was unable to communicate with those who visited us. Many times, I was unable to open my eyes, speak, or move. Some people would enter the hospital room, start talking with DeeDee as though I were not in the room, and, often, negative words would flow out of their mouths. I could hear everything they said!

Look how bad he looks. Look at all of those machines. Does Carl know how bad he is doing? What are you going to do with Carl? Do you think he will get better? Look at all those tubes and machines Carl is hooked up to! How do you stay here with him? If I were you, DeeDee...

I wanted to throw the people out of the room if I could!

When someone cannot communicate, it does not mean they cannot hear everything in the hospital room. When you make a hospital visit, prepare yourself to see a person who you have never seen in a hospital gown and hooked up to tubes, machines, and an oxygen mask.

At Home:

Please keep things positive. Do not start the conversation with, "How are you doing?" Instead, start with something positive! Ask them if they are comfortable or if it is a good time for them. Offer to help however you can, which can look like: bringing in their mail, taking out the garbage, washing dishes, or running an errand.

You can also ask if you can get them anything or help another way. Find ways to help the person!

Before You Leave:

There are many ways to end a visit, but my first recommendation is to pray for them. Ask God to heal and restore them to perfect health!

Other things you can do are share scripture with them, continue to lift them up to the Lord in your personal prayer time, or offer to help them with something!

CHAPTER 21
A GUIDE TO HOSPITAL AND HOME VISITS

"Therefore, as we have opportunity, let us do good to all people, especially to those who belong to the family of believers."
(Galatians 6:10 NIV)

There are many things to consider when visiting someone in the hospital. Here are some helpful suggestions for how to conduct yourself for effective ministry during a visit!

In The Hospital:

Please, above all else, be positive in your words and comments. Be an encouragement to the patient and their loved ones who are present! Ask if this is a good time to make a short visit, and keep your visit short—ten to fifteen minutes at the most. If a doctor, nurse, or medical personnel enters the room, please excuse yourself from the room until they are finished with their business or task. Many times in the medical community, they do not stop and ask how well you know the patient before asking personal questions. The patient may not be comfortable answering with you in the room!

Keep your visit short and encouraging. Ask their loved ones if you can pick them up something to eat. Ask if you can help them while they are at the hospital caring for a loved one.

Please remember to pray with the patient before you leave. Sing a song of praise and worship or a hymn. Pray the Lord's Prayer or read scriptures to them.

Tips for a Successful Home Visit:

Again, please keep things positive! Keep the visit short, unless you are helping them with tasks around the house. Always ask if it is a good time to visit.

Look for things that you can do to help the person as they recover. If the trash can is full, empty it. If they are out of facial tissues or paper towels, go get some for them. Ask them if they would like something to drink, if you can pick them up something, or if they'd like you to make them something to eat.

Note: Please ask if they are sleeping well. Many people need to sleep in recliners after surgeries. If they don't have one, find one for them!

Before You Leave:

As always, pray for them. Ask God to heal and restore them to perfect health!

CHAPTER 22
WHAT YOU CAN DO TO HELP!

"Be devoted to one another in love. Honor one another above yourselves."
(Romans 12:10 NIV)

t's hard enough to take care of someone with poor health, let alone take care of the daily needs around the home. If you want to help others in home-bound care, here are some practical ways that you can make a difference!

Help Around the House:

- Mow the lawn, plant flowers, rake leaves, or shovel snow
- Clean out gutters, wash windows, touch up, or paint
- Set up or tear down outdoor holiday decorations
- Build a wheelchair ramp or add railings to both sides of stairs

- Clean and organize the garage, carport, or basement
- Organize medications and supplies
- Organize kitchen cabinets and pantries
- Organize bedroom and hall closets
- Clean the refrigerator and oven
- Wash and vacuum the floors
- Wash sheets, linens, and clothes
- Prepare easy-to-cook meals
- Clean bathrooms
- Dust the house and change burned-out light bulbs
- Go shopping for them or run errands

Help with Transportation:

- To and from the hospital
- To doctor, dental, or other medical appointments
- To shop at the grocery store, drug store, post office, or somewhere else
- To church, support groups, restaurants, or meetings

Helpful Personal Care:

- Read healing scriptures to them
- Read poems or short stories
- Play musical instruments or sing music
- Write thank you notes or letters for them
- Answer their voicemails and emails
- Update their CaringBridge site
- Write checks for their bills and mail them

Other Helpful Things to Consider:

- Pray for them and share prayer requests with others
- Read and leave a scripture verse with them
- Continue to lift them up to the Lord and help them
- Communicate with family members who are out of state

Above all else—whether you help daily, weekly, monthly, quarterly, or once a year—please do so without complaining. The person who needs help wants to be encouraged and built up! THANK YOU!

HEALING SCRIPTURES FROM GOD'S WORD

The following scriptures are taken from the New International Version (NIV). They have brought us comfort and encouragement over the past twenty years with our struggles with major health problems in my life.

"In the beginning God created the heavens and the earth."
(Genesis 1:1)

"I will make you into a great nation, and I will bless you."
(Genesis 12:3)

"For I am the Lord, who heals you."
(Exodus 15:26)

"The Lord bless you and keep you; the Lord make his face shine on you and be gracious to you; the Lord turn his face toward you and give you peace."'
(Numbers 6:24-26)

"When a man makes a vow to the Lord or takes an oath to

obligate himself by a pledge, he must not break his word but
must do everything he said."
(Numbers 30:2)

"What other nation is so great as to have their gods near them
the way the Lord our God is near us whenever we pray to
him?"
(Deuteronomy 4:7)

"Be careful to obey so that it may go well with you and that
you may increase greatly."
(Deuteronomy 6:3)

"Hear, O Israel: The Lord our God, the Lord is one. Love the
Lord your God with all your heart and with all your soul and
with all your strength."
(Deuteronomy 6:4-5)

"Be careful that you do not forget the Lord, who brought you
out of Egypt, out of the land of slavery."
(Deuteronomy 6:12)

"Love the Lord your God and to serve him with all your heart
and with all your soul."
(Deuteronomy 11:13)

"For the Lord your God will bless you in all your harvest and
in all the work of your hands, and your joy will be complete."
(Deuteronomy 16:15)

"And when you and your children return to the Lord your
God and obey him with all your heart and with all your soul
according to everything I command you today, then the Lord

your God will restore your fortunes and have compassion on
you."
(Deuteronomy 30:2-3)

"Now choose life, so that you and your children may live and
that you may love the Lord your God."
(Deuteronomy 30:19-20)

"The Lord himself goes before you and will be with you; he
will never leave you nor forsake you. Do not be afraid; do not
be discouraged."
(Deuteronomy 31:8)

"Have I not commanded you? Be strong and courageous. Do
not be afraid; do not be discouraged, for the Lord your God
will be with you wherever you go."
(Joshua 1:9)

"Joshua said to them, 'Do not be afraid; do not be
discouraged. Be strong and courageous. This is what the Lord
will do to all the enemies you are going to fight.'"
(Joshua 10:25)

"Be very strong; be careful to obey all that is written in the
Book of the Law of Moses, without turning aside to the right
or to the left."
(Joshua 23:6)

"The Lord does not look at the things people look at. People
look at the outward appearance, but the Lord looks at the
heart."
(1 Samuel 16:7)

"Long life to you! Good health to you and your household!
And good health to all that is yours!"
(1 Samuel 25:6)

"I have heard your prayer and seen your tears; I will heal
you."
(2 Kings 20:5)

"For the Lord searches every heart and understands every
desire and every thought."
(1 Chronicles 28:9)

"David also said to Solomon his son, 'Be strong and
courageous, and do the work. Do not be afraid or
discouraged, for the Lord God, my God, is with you. He will
not fail you or forsake you…'"
(1 Chronicles 28:20)

"If my people, who are called by my name, will humble
themselves and pray and seek my face and turn from their
wicked ways, then I will hear from heaven, and I will forgive
their sin and will heal their land."
(2 Chronicles 7:14)

"The priests and the Levites stood to bless the people, and
God heard them, for their prayer reached heaven, his holy
dwelling place."
(2 Chronicles 30:27)

"Lord, let your ear be attentive to the prayer of this your
servant and to the prayer of your servants who delight in
revering your name. Give your servant success today by
granting him favor in the presence of this man."
(Nehemiah 1:11)

"This day is holy to our Lord. Do not grieve, for the joy of the
Lord is your strength."
(Nehemiah 8:10)

"Naked I came from my mother's womb, and naked I will
depart. The LORD gave and the LORD has taken away; may
the name of the LORD be praised."
(Job 1:21)

"The Spirit of God has made me; the breath of the Almighty
gives me life."
(Job 33:4)

"The Lord has heard my cry for mercy; the Lord accepts my
prayer."
(Psalm 6:9)

"The Lord is a refuge for the oppressed, a stronghold in times
of trouble."
(Psalm 9:9)

"You, Lord, hear the desire of the afflicted; you encourage
them, and you listen to their cry."
(Psalm 10:17)

"The heavens declare the glory of God; the skies proclaim the
work of his hands. Day after day they pour forth speech;
night after night they reveal knowledge. They have no
speech, they use no words; no sound is heard from them. Yet
their voice goes out into all the earth, their words to the ends
of the world."
(Psalm 19:1-4)

"May these words of my mouth and this meditation of my

heart be pleasing in your sight, Lord, my Rock and my
Redeemer."
(Psalm 19:14)

"May he give you the desire of your heart and make all your
plans succeed."
(Psalm 20:4)

"To you they cried out and were saved; in you they trusted
and were not put to shame."
(Psalm 22:5)

"Even though I walk through the darkest valley, I will fear no
evil, for you are with me; your rod and your staff, they
comfort me."
(Psalm 23:4)

"He guides the humble in what is right and teaches them his
way."
(Psalm 25:9)

"The Lord is my light and my salvation—whom shall I fear?
The Lord is the stronghold of my life—of whom shall I be
afraid?"
(Psalm 27:1)

"For in the day of trouble he will keep me safe in his
dwelling."
(Psalm 27:5)

"You are my hiding place; you will protect me from trouble
and surround me with songs of deliverance."
(Psalm 32:7)

"Take delight in the Lord, and he will give you the desires of
your heart."
(Psalm 37:4)

"But now, Lord, what do I look for? My hope is in you."
(Psalm 39:7)

"Blessed are those who have regard for the weak; the Lord
delivers them in times of trouble."
(Psalm 41:1)

"I said, 'Have mercy on me, Lord; heal me, for I have sinned
against you.'"
(Psalm 41:4)

"Then I will go to the altar of God, to God, my joy and my
delight. I will praise you with the lyre, O God, my God."
(Psalm 43:4)

"God is our refuge and strength, an ever-present help in
trouble."
(Psalm 46:1)

"Call on me in the day of trouble; I will deliver you, and you
will honor me."
(Psalm 50:15)

"Have mercy on me, O God, according to your unfailing love;
according to your great compassion blot out my transgressions.
Wash away all my iniquity and cleanse me from my sin."
(Psalm 51:1-2)

"Create in me a pure heart, O God, and renew a steadfast

spirit within me. Do not cast me from your presence or take your Holy Spirit from me. Restore to me the joy of your salvation and grant me a willing spirit, to sustain me."
(Psalm 51:10-12)

"Cast your cares on the Lord and he will sustain you; he will never let the righteous be shaken."
(Psalm 55:22)

"Shout for joy to God, all the earth!"
(Psalm 66:1)

"May people ever pray for him and bless him all day long."
(Psalm 72:15)

"Blessed are those whose strength is in you."
(Psalm 84:5)

"Hear my prayer, Lord; listen to my cry for mercy."
(Psalm 86:6)

"With long life I will satisfy him and show him my salvation."
(Psalm 91:16)

"Praise the Lord, my soul; all my inmost being, praise his holy name."
(Psalm 103:1)

"Who forgives all your sins and heals all your diseases."
(Psalm 103:3)

"How many are your works, Lord! In wisdom you made them all; the earth is full of your creatures."

(Psalm 104:24)

"Praise the Lord. Blessed are those who fear the Lord, who find great delight in his commands."
(Psalm 112:1)

"Their righteousness endures forever..."
(Psalm 112:9)

"Precious in the sight of the Lord is the death of his faithful servants."
(Psalm 116:15)

"The Lord is with me; I will not be afraid. What can mere mortals do to me? The Lord is with me; he is my helper. I look in triumph on my enemies."
(Psalm 118:6-7)

"I am laid low in the dust; preserve my life according to your word."
(Psalm 119:25)

"Give me understanding, so that I may keep your law and obey it with all my heart."
(Psalm 119:34)

"Your word is a lamp for my feet, a light on my path."
(Psalm 119:105)

"I lift up my eyes to the mountains—where does my help come from? My help comes from the Lord, the Maker of heaven and earth. He will not let your foot slip—he who watches over you will not slumber; indeed, he who watches over Israel will neither slumber nor sleep. The Lord watches

over you—the Lord is your shade at your right hand; the sun will not harm you by day, nor the moon by night. The Lord will keep you from all harm—he will watch over your life; the Lord will watch over your coming and going both now and forevermore."
(Psalm 121:1-8)

"Give thanks to the Lord, for he is good. *His love endures forever.*"
(Psalm 136:1)

"Set a guard over my mouth, Lord; keep watch over the door of my lips."
(Psalm 141:3)

"He heals the brokenhearted and binds up their wounds."
(Psalm 147:3)

"Praise the Lord. Praise God in his sanctuary; praise him in his mighty heavens. Praise him for his acts of power; praise him for his surpassing greatness. Praise him with the sounding of the trumpet, praise him with the harp and lyre, praise him with timbrel and dancing, praise him with the strings and pipe, praise him with the clash of cymbals, praise him with resounding cymbals. Let everything that has breath praise the Lord. Praise the Lord."
(Psalm 150:1-6)

"Then you will win favor and a good name in the sight of God and man."
(Proverbs 3:4)

"Trust in the Lord with all your heart and lean not on your

own understanding; in all your ways submit to him, and he
will make your paths straight."
(Proverbs 3:5-6)

"This will bring health to your body and nourishment to your
bones."
(Proverbs 3:8)

"Blessed are those who find wisdom, those who gain
understanding."
(Proverbs 3:13)

"He mocks proud mockers but shows favor to the humble
and oppressed."
(Proverbs 3:34)

"For they are life to those who find them and health to one's
whole body."
(Proverbs 4:22)

"Blessings crown the head of the righteous…"
(Proverbs 10:6)

"The fear of the Lord adds length to life…"
(Proverbs 10:27)

"Evildoers are trapped by their sinful talk, and so the
innocent escape trouble."
(Proverbs 12:13)

"The Lord detests the sacrifice of the wicked, but the prayer
of the upright pleases him."
(Proverbs 15:8)

"Light in a messenger's eyes brings joy to the heart, and good news gives health to the bones."
(Proverbs 15:30)

"A faithful person will be richly blessed, but one eager to get rich will not go unpunished."
(Proverbs 28:20)

"Charm is deceptive, and beauty is fleeting; but a woman who fears the Lord is to be praised."
(Proverbs 31:30)

"I know that everything God does will endure forever."
(Ecclesiastes 3:14)

"Whatever your hand finds to do, do it with all your might."
(Ecclesiastes 9:10)

"Remember your Creator in the days of your youth, before the days of trouble come."
(Ecclesiastes 12:1)

"Let him lead me to the banquet hall, and let his banner over me be love."
(Song Of Songs 2:4)

"See, I lay a stone in Zion, a tested stone, a precious cornerstone for a sure foundation; the one who relies on it will never be stricken with panic."
(Isaiah 28:16)

"They will enter Zion with singing; everlasting joy will crown their heads. Gladness and joy will overtake them, and sorrow and sighing will flee away."

(Isaiah 35:10)

"Lord, by such things people live; and my spirit finds life in them too. You restored me to health and let me live."
(Isaiah 38:16)

"So do not fear, for I am with you; do not be dismayed, for I am your God. I will strengthen you and help you; I will uphold you with my righteous right hand."
(Isaiah 41:10)

"He will not falter or be discouraged till he establishes justice on earth."
(Isaiah 42:4)

"The Lord is the everlasting God, the Creator of the ends of the earth. He will not grow tired or weary, and his understanding no one can fathom. He gives strength to the weary and increases the power of the weak. Even youths grow tired and weary, and young men stumble and fall; but those who hope in the Lord will renew their strength. They will soar on wings like eagles; they will run and not grow weary, they will walk and not be faint."
(Isaiah 40:28-31)

"So do not fear, for I am with you; do not be dismayed, for I am your God. I will strengthen you and help you; I will uphold you with my righteous right hand."
(Isaiah 41:10)

"For I am the Lord your God who takes hold of your right hand and says to you, Do not fear; I will help you."
(Isaiah 41:13)

"But he was pierced for our transgressions, he was crushed for our iniquities; the punishment that brought us peace was on him, and by his wounds we are healed."
(Isaiah 53:5)

"You will go out in joy and be led forth in peace; the mountains and hills will burst into song before you, and all the trees of the field will clap their hands."
(Isaiah 55:12)

"And I will heal them."
(Isaiah 57:19)

"Then your light will break forth like the dawn, and your healing will quickly appear; then your righteousness will go before you, and the glory of the Lord will be your rear guard."
(Isaiah 58:8)

"Then you will call, and the Lord will answer; you will cry for help, and he will say: Here am I."
(Isaiah 58:9)

"These are the ones I look on with favor: those who are humble and contrite in spirit, and who tremble at my word."
(Isaiah 66:2)

"Lord, I know that people's lives are not their own; it is not for them to direct their steps."
(Jeremiah 10:23)

"But I will restore you to health and heal your wounds."
(Jeremiah 30:17)

"Ah, Sovereign Lord, you have made the heavens and the earth by your great power and outstretched arm. Nothing is too hard for you."
(Jeremiah 32:17)

"Nevertheless, I will bring health and healing to it; I will heal my people and will let them enjoy abundant peace and security."
(Jeremiah 33:6)

"Yet this I call to mind and therefore I have hope: Because of the Lord's great love we are not consumed, for his compassions never fail. They are new every morning; great is your faithfulness. I say to myself, 'The Lord is my portion; therefore I will wait for him.' The Lord is good to those whose hope is in him, to the one who seeks him."
(Lamentations 3:21-25)

"Praise be to the name of God for ever and ever; wisdom and power are his. He changes times and seasons; he deposes kings and raises up others. He gives wisdom to the wise and knowledge to the discerning. He reveals deep and hidden things; he knows what lies in darkness, and light dwells with him. I thank and praise you, God of my ancestors: You have given me wisdom and power, you have made known to me what we asked of you, you have made known to us the dream of the king."
(Daniel 2:20-23)

"I will make them and the places surrounding my hill a blessing. I will send down showers in season; there will be showers of blessing."
(Ezekiel 34:26)

"The Lord is good, a refuge in times of trouble. He cares for those who trust in him."
(Nahum 1:7)

"'Not by might nor by power, but by my Spirit,' says the Lord Almighty."
(Zechariah 4:6)

"And when you pray, do not be like the hypocrites, for they love to pray standing in the synagogues and on the street corners to be seen by others. Truly I tell you, they have received their reward in full."
(Matthew 6:5)

"Therefore I tell you, do not worry about your life, what you will eat or drink; or about your body, what you will wear. Is not life more than food, and the body more than clothes?"
(Matthew 6:25)

"Can any one of you by worrying add a single hour to your life? "And why do you worry about clothes? See how the flowers of the field grow. They do not labor or spin."
(Matthew 6:27-28)

"So do not worry, saying, 'What shall we eat?' or 'What shall we drink?' or 'What shall we wear?'"
(Matthew 6:31)

"Therefore do not worry about tomorrow, for tomorrow will worry about itself. Each day has enough trouble of its own."
(Matthew 6:34)

"Jesus turned and saw her. 'Take heart, daughter,' he said,

'your faith has healed you.' And the woman was healed at
that moment."
(Matthew 9:22)

"Heal the sick, raise the dead, cleanse those who have
leprosy, drive out demons. Freely you have received; freely
give."
(Matthew 10:8)

"But when they arrest you, do not worry about what to say or
how to say it. At that time you will be given what to say."
(Matthew 10:19)

"The blind receive sight…"
(Matthew 11:5)

"Come to me, all you who are weary and burdened, and I
will give you rest. Take my yoke upon you and learn from
me, for I am gentle and humble in heart, and you will find
rest for your souls."
(Matthew 11:28-29)

"Make a tree good and its fruit will be good, or make a tree
bad and its fruit will be bad, for a tree is recognized by its
fruit."
(Matthew 12:33)

"But I tell you that everyone will have to give account on the
day of judgment for every empty word they have spoken."
(Matthew 12:36)

"Therefore, whoever takes the lowly position of this child is
the greatest in the kingdom of heaven."
(Matthew 18:4)

"See that you do not despise one of these little ones. For I tell
you that their angels in heaven always see the face of my
Father in heaven."
(Matthew 18:10-11)

"'Haven't you read,' he replied, 'that at the beginning the
Creator made them male and female...'"
(Matthew 19:4)

"For those who exalt themselves will be humbled, and those
who humble themselves will be exalted."
(Matthew 23:12)

"I was sick and you looked after me."
(Matthew 25:36)

"On hearing this, Jesus said to them, 'It is not the healthy who
need a doctor, but the sick. I have not come to call the
righteous, but sinners.'"
(Mark 2:17)

"With man this is impossible, but not with God; all things are
possible with God."
(Mark 10:27)

"'Go,' said Jesus, 'your faith has healed you.' Immediately he
received his sight and followed Jesus along the road."
(Mark 10:52)

"Therefore I tell you, whatever you ask for in prayer, believe
that you have received it, and it will be yours."
(Mark 11:24)

"Jesus answered them, 'It is not the healthy who need a
doctor, but the sick.'"
(Luke 5:31)

"But to you who are listening I say: Love your enemies, do
good to those who hate you, bless those who curse you, pray
for those who mistreat you."
(Luke 6:27-28)

"And a woman was there who had been subject to bleeding
for twelve years, but no one could heal her."
(Luke 8:43)

"Then he said to her, 'Daughter, your faith has healed you. Go
in peace.'"
(Luke 8:48)

"Hearing this, Jesus said to Jairus, 'Don't be afraid; just
believe, and she will be healed.'"
(Luke 8:50)

"He went to him and bandaged his wounds, pouring on oil
and wine. Then he put the man on his own donkey, brought
him to an inn and took care of him."
(Luke 10:34)

"Then Jesus said to his disciples: 'Therefore I tell you, do not
worry about your life, what you will eat; or about your body,
what you will wear.'"
(Luke 12:22a)

"In the beginning was the Word, and the Word was with God,
and the Word was God. He was with God in the beginning.

Through him all things were made; without him nothing was made that has been made. In him was life, and that life was the light of all mankind. The light shines in the darkness, and the darkness has not overcome it."
(John 1:1-5)

"For God so loved the world that he gave his one and only Son, that whoever believes in him shall not perish but have eternal life. For God did not send his Son into the world to condemn the world, but to save the world through him."
(John 3:16-17)

"Then Jesus declared, 'I am the bread of life. Whoever comes to me will never go hungry, and whoever believes in me will never be thirsty.'"
(John 6:35)

"I am the gate; whoever enters through me will be saved. They will come in and go out, and find pasture. The thief comes only to steal and kill and destroy; I have come that they may have life, and have it to the full. I am the good shepherd. The good shepherd lays down his life for the sheep."
(John 10:9-11)

"Jesus said to her, 'I am the resurrection and the life. The one who believes in me will live, even though they die; and whoever lives by believing in me will never die. Do you believe this?'"
(John 11:25-26)

"A new command I give you: Love one another. As I have loved you, so you must love one another. By this everyone will know that you are my disciples, if you love one another."

(John 13:34-35)

"Do not let your hearts be troubled. You believe in God; believe also in me. My Father's house has many rooms; if that were not so, would I have told you that I am going there to prepare a place for you? And if I go and prepare a place for you, I will come back and take you to be with me that you also may be where I am. You know the way to the place where I am going."
(John 14:1-4)

"Jesus answered, 'I am the way and the truth and the life. No one comes to the Father except through me.'"
(John 14:6)

"Jesus replied, 'Anyone who loves me will obey my teaching. My Father will love them, and we will come to them and make our home with them.'"
(John 14:23)

"Peace I leave with you; my peace I give you. I do not give to you as the world gives. Do not let your hearts be troubled and do not be afraid."
(John 14:27)

"I have told you this so that my joy may be in you and that your joy may be complete."
(John 15:11)

"Greater love has no one than this: to lay down one's life for one's friends."
(John 15:13)

"In this world you will have trouble. But take heart! I have
overcome the world."
(John 16:33)

"Remain in me, as I also remain in you."
(John 15:4)

"Again Jesus said, 'Simon son of John, do you love me?' He
answered, 'Yes, Lord, you know that I love you.' Jesus said,
'Take care of my sheep.'"
(John 21:16)

"Peter and the other apostles replied: 'We must obey God
rather than human beings!'"
(Acts 5:29)

"Judas and Silas, who themselves were prophets, said much
to encourage and strengthen the believers."
(Acts 15:32)

"In everything I did, I showed you that by this kind of hard
work we must help the weak, remembering the words the
Lord Jesus himself said: 'It is more blessed to give than to
receive.'"
(Acts 20:35)

"But God has helped me to this very day; so I stand here and
testify to small and great alike."
(Acts 26:22)

"Through him we received grace and apostleship to call all
the Gentiles to the obedience that comes from faith for his
name's sake."
(Romans 1:5)

"For I am not ashamed of the gospel, because it is the power of God that brings salvation to everyone who believes: first to the Jew, then to the Gentile."
(Romans 1:16)

"They exchanged the truth about God for a lie, and worshiped and served created things rather than the Creator —who is forever praised. Amen."
(Romans 1:25)

"For God does not show favoritism."
(Romans 2:11)

"For all have sinned and fall short of the glory of God."
(Romans 3:23)

"Blessed is the one whose sin the Lord will never count against them."
(Romans 4:8)

"And hope does not put us to shame, because God's love has been poured out into our hearts through the Holy Spirit, who has been given to us."
(Romans 5:5)

"But God demonstrates his own love for us in this: While we were still sinners, Christ died for us."
(Romans 5:8)

"In the same way, count yourselves dead to sin but alive to God in Christ Jesus."
(Romans 6:11)

"Do not offer any part of yourself to sin as an instrument of

wickedness, but rather offer yourselves to God as those who have been brought from death to life; and offer every part of yourself to him as an instrument of righteousness."
(Romans 6:13)

"Don't you know that when you offer yourselves to someone as obedient slaves, you are slaves of the one you obey— whether you are slaves to sin, which leads to death, or to obedience, which leads to righteousness?"
(Romans 6:16)

"For the wages of sin is death, but the gift of God is eternal life in Christ Jesus our Lord."
(Romans 6:23)

"In the same way, the Spirit helps us in our weakness. We do not know what we ought to pray for, but the Spirit himself intercedes for us through wordless groans."
(Romans 8:26)

"And we know that in all things God works for the good of those who love him, who have been called according to his purpose."
(Romans 8:28)

"What, then, shall we say in response to these things? If God is for us, who can be against us? He who did not spare his own Son, but gave him up for us all—how will he not also, along with him, graciously give us all things? Who will bring any charge against those whom God has chosen? It is God who justifies. Who then is the one who condemns? No one. Christ Jesus who died—more than that, who was raised to life —is at the right hand of God and is also interceding for us."
(Romans 8:31-34)

"Who shall separate us from the love of Christ? Shall trouble or hardship or persecution or famine or nakedness or danger or sword? As it is written: 'For your sake we face death all day long; we are considered as sheep to be slaughtered.' No, in all these things we are more than conquerors through him who loved us. For I am convinced that neither death nor life, neither angels nor demons, neither the present nor the future, nor any powers, neither height nor depth, nor anything else in all creation, will be able to separate us from the love of God that is in Christ Jesus our Lord."
(Romans 8:35-39)

"If you declare with your mouth, 'Jesus is Lord,' and believe in your heart that God raised him from the dead, you will be saved. For it is with your heart that you believe and are justified, and it is with your mouth that you profess your faith and are saved."
(Romans 10:9-10)

"For there is no difference between Jew and Gentile—the same Lord is Lord of all and richly blesses all who call on him, for, 'Everyone who calls on the name of the Lord will be saved.'"
(Romans 10:12-13)

"For God's gifts and his call are irrevocable."
(Romans 11:29)

"Therefore, I urge you, brothers and sisters, in view of God's mercy, to offer your bodies as a living sacrifice, holy and pleasing to God—this is your true and proper worship."
(Romans 12:1)

"If it is to encourage, then give encouragement; if it is giving,

then give generously; if it is to lead, do it diligently; if it is to show mercy, do it cheerfully."
(Romans 12:8)

"Love must be sincere. Hate what is evil; cling to what is good."
(Romans 12:9)

"Be devoted to one another in love. Honor one another above yourselves."
(Romans 12:10)

"Be joyful in hope, patient in affliction, faithful in prayer."
(Romans 12:12)

"Share with the Lord's people who are in need. Practice hospitality."
(Romans 12:13)

"Do not repay anyone evil for evil. Be careful to do what is right in the eyes of everyone."
(Romans 12:17)

"So then, each of us will give an account of ourselves to God."
(Romans 14:12)

"Accept one another, then, just as Christ accepted you, in order to bring praise to God."
(Romans 15:7)

"May the God of hope fill you with all joy and peace as you trust in him, so that you may overflow with hope by the power of the Holy Spirit."

(Romans 15:13)

"Do you not know that your bodies are temples of the Holy Spirit, who is in you, whom you have received from God? You are not your own; you were bought at a price. Therefore honor God with your bodies."
(1 Corinthians 6:19-20)

"It is sown a natural body, it is raised a spiritual body. If there is a natural body, there is also a spiritual body."
(1 Corinthians 15:44)

"But thanks be to God! He gives us the victory through our Lord Jesus Christ."
(1 Corinthians 15:57)

"For we live by faith, not by sight."
(2 Corinthians 5:7)

"Therefore, if anyone is in Christ, the new creation has come: The old has gone, the new is here!"
(2 Corinthians 5:17)

"I have spoken to you with great frankness; I take great pride in you. I am greatly encouraged; in all our troubles my joy knows no bounds."
(2 Corinthians 7:4)

"For I know your eagerness to help, and I have been boasting about it…"
(2 Corinthians 9:2)

"But the fruit of the Spirit is love, joy, peace, forbearance, kindness, goodness, faithfulness, gentleness and self-control.

Against such things there is no law. Those who belong to
Christ Jesus have crucified the flesh with its passions and
desires. Since we live by the Spirit, let us keep in step with the
Spirit."
(Galatians 5:22-25)

"Let us not become weary in doing good, for at the proper
time we will reap a harvest if we do not give up."
(Galatians 6:9)

"Neither circumcision nor uncircumcision means anything;
what counts is the new creation."
(Galatians 6:15)

"But because of his great love for us, God, who is rich in
mercy, made us alive with Christ even when we were dead in
transgressions—it is by grace you have been saved. And God
raised us up with Christ and seated us with him in the
heavenly realms in Christ Jesus."
(Ephesians 2:4-6)

"For it is by grace you have been saved, through faith—and
this is not from yourselves, it is the gift of God—not by
works, so that no one can boast."
(Ephesians 2:8-9)

"In him and through faith in him we may approach God with
freedom and confidence."
(Ephesians 3:12)

"Now to him who is able to do immeasurably more than all
we ask or imagine, according to his power that is at work
within us."
(Ephesians 3:20)

"Do not let any unwholesome talk come out of your mouths, but only what is helpful for building others up according to their needs, that it may benefit those who listen."
(Ephesians 4:29)

"Be kind and compassionate to one another, forgiving each other, just as in Christ God forgave you."
(Ephesians 4:32)

"Follow God's example, therefore, as dearly loved children and walk in the way of love, just as Christ loved us and gave himself up for us as a fragrant offering and sacrifice to God."
(Ephesians 5:1-2)

"For you were once darkness, but now you are light in the Lord. Live as children of light."
(Ephesians 5:8)

"Have nothing to do with the fruitless deeds of darkness, but rather expose them. It is shameful even to mention what the disobedient do in secret."
(Ephesians 5:11-12)

"Submit to one another out of reverence for Christ."
(Ephesians 5:21)

"After all, no one ever hated their own body, but they feed and care for their body, just as Christ does the church."
(Ephesians 5:29)

"Finally, be strong in the Lord and in his mighty power. Put on the full armor of God, so that you can take your stand against the devil's schemes."
(Ephesians 6:10-11)

"...being confident of this, that he who began a good work in you will carry it on to completion until the day of Christ Jesus."
(Philippians 1:6)

"I eagerly expect and hope that I will in no way be ashamed, but will have sufficient courage so that now as always Christ will be exalted in my body, whether by life or by death."
(Philippians 1:20)

"For to me, to live is Christ and to die is gain."
(Philippians 1:21)

"In your relationships with one another, have the same mindset as Christ Jesus."
(Philippians 2:5)

"And being found in appearance as a man, he humbled himself by becoming obedient to death—even death on a cross! Therefore God exalted him to the highest place and gave him the name that is above every name, that at the name of Jesus every knee should bow, in heaven and on earth and under the earth, and every tongue acknowledge that Jesus Christ is Lord, to the glory of God the Father."
(Philippians 2:8-11)

"Do everything without grumbling or arguing."
(Philippians 2:14)

"But our citizenship is in heaven. And we eagerly await a Savior from there, the Lord Jesus Christ, who, by the power that enables him to bring everything under his control, will transform our lowly bodies so that they will be like his glorious body."

(Philippians 3:20-21)

"Rejoice in the Lord always. I will say it again: Rejoice!"
(Philippians 4:4)

"Do not be anxious about anything, but in every situation, by prayer and petition, with thanksgiving, present your requests to God. And the peace of God, which transcends all understanding, will guard your hearts and your minds in Christ Jesus. Finally, brothers and sisters, whatever is true, whatever is noble, whatever is right, whatever is pure, whatever is lovely, whatever is admirable—if anything is excellent or praiseworthy—think about such things."
(Philippians 4:6-8)

"I can do all this through him who gives me strength."
(Philippians 4:13)

"Set your minds on things above, not on earthly things. For you died, and your life is now hidden with Christ in God. When Christ, who is your life, appears, then you also will appear with him in glory."
(Colossians 3:2-4)

"...and have put on the new self, which is being renewed in knowledge in the image of its Creator."
(Colossians 3:10)

"Bear with each other and forgive one another if any of you has a grievance against someone. Forgive as the Lord forgave you."
(Colossians 3:13)

"Therefore encourage one another with these words."

(1 Thessalonians 4:18)

"And is well known for her good deeds, such as bringing up children, showing hospitality, washing the feet of the Lord's people, helping those in trouble and devoting herself to all kinds of good deeds."
(1 Timothy 5:10)

"All Scripture is God-breathed and is useful for teaching, rebuking, correcting and training in righteousness, so that the servant of God may be thoroughly equipped for every good work."
(2 Timothy 3:16-17)

"But encourage one another daily, as long as it is called 'Today,' so that none of you may be hardened by sin's deceitfulness."
(Hebrews 3:13)

"For the word of God is alive and active. Sharper than any double-edged sword, it penetrates even to dividing soul and spirit, joints and marrow; it judges the thoughts and attitudes of the heart."
(Hebrews 4:12)

"...not giving up meeting together, as some are in the habit of doing, but encouraging one another—and all the more as you see the Day approaching."
(Hebrews 10:25)

"Now faith is confidence in what we hope for and assurance about what we do not see."
(Hebrews 11:1)

"And without faith it is impossible to please God, because anyone who comes to him must believe that he exists and that he rewards those who earnestly seek him."
(Hebrews 11:6)

"Therefore, since we are surrounded by such a great cloud of witnesses, let us throw off everything that hinders and the sin that so easily entangles. And let us run with perseverance the race marked out for us, fixing our eyes on Jesus, the pioneer and perfecter of faith. For the joy set before him he endured the cross, scorning its shame, and sat down at the right hand of the throne of God. Consider him who endured such opposition from sinners, so that you will not grow weary and lose heart."
(Hebrews 12:1-3)

"Endure hardship as discipline; God is treating you as his children. For what children are not disciplined by their father?"
(Hebrews 12:7)

"Keep your lives free from the love of money and be content with what you have, because God has said, 'Never will I leave you; never will I forsake you.'"
(Hebrews 13:5)

"Consider it pure joy, my brothers and sisters, whenever you face trials of many kinds."
(James 1:2)

"Blessed is the one who perseveres under trial because, having stood the test, that person will receive the crown of life that the Lord has promised to those who love him."
(James 1:12)

"Do not merely listen to the word, and so deceive yourselves. Do what it says. Anyone who listens to the word but does not do what it says is like someone who looks at his face in a mirror and, after looking at himself, goes away and immediately forgets what he looks like. But whoever looks intently into the perfect law that gives freedom, and continues in it—not forgetting what they have heard, but doing it—they will be blessed in what they do."
(James 1:22-25)

"Out of the same mouth come praise and cursing. My brothers and sisters, this should not be."
(James 3:10)

"Humble yourselves before the Lord, and he will lift you up."
(James 4:10)

"Is anyone among you in trouble? Let them pray."
(James 5:13)

"And the prayer offered in faith will make the sick person well; the Lord will raise them up. If they have sinned, they will be forgiven."
(James 5:15)

"The prayer of a righteous person is powerful and effective."
(James 5:16)

"He was chosen before the creation of the world, but was revealed in these last times for your sake."
(1 Peter 1:20)

"Rather, it should be that of your inner self, the unfading

beauty of a gentle and quiet spirit, which is of great worth in
God's sight."
(1 Peter 3:4)

"Husbands, in the same way be considerate as you live with
your wives, and treat them with respect as the weaker partner
and as heirs with you of the gracious gift of life, so that
nothing will hinder your prayers."
(1 Peter 3:7)

"For the eyes of the Lord are on the righteous and his ears are
attentive to their prayer."
(1 Peter 3:12)

"Dear friends, do not be surprised at the fiery ordeal that has
come on you to test you, as though something strange were
happening to you."
(1 Peter 4:12)

"So then, those who suffer according to God's will should
commit themselves to their faithful Creator and continue to
do good."
(1 Peter 4:19)

"Be shepherds of God's flock that is under your care,
watching over them—not because you must, but because you
are willing, as God wants you to be."
(1 Peter 5:2)

"Cast all your anxiety on him because he cares for you."
(1 Peter 5:7)

"The Lord is not slow in keeping his promise, as some
understand slowness."

(2 Peter 3:9)

"But in keeping with his promise we are looking forward to a new heaven and a new earth, where righteousness dwells. So then, dear friends, since you are looking forward to this, make every effort to be found spotless, blameless and at peace with him."
(2 Peter 3:13-14)

"My dear children, I write this to you so that you will not sin. But if anybody does sin, we have an advocate with the Father —Jesus Christ, the Righteous One. He is the atoning sacrifice for our sins, and not only for ours but also for the sins of the whole world. We know that we have come to know him if we keep his commands."
(1 John 2:1-3)

"And this is what he promised us—eternal life."
(1 John 2:25)

"This is how we know what love is: Jesus Christ laid down his life for us. And we ought to lay down our lives for our brothers and sisters."
(1 John 3:16)

"You, dear children, are from God and have overcome them, because the one who is in you is greater than the one who is in the world."
(1 John 4:4)

"And this is the testimony: God has given us eternal life, and this life is in his Son."
(1 John 5:11)

"And this is love: that we walk in obedience to his
commands. As you have heard from the beginning, his
command is that you walk in love."
(2 John 6)

"Dear friend, I pray that you may enjoy good health and that all
may go well with you, even as your soul is getting along well."
(3 John 2)

"You have persevered and have endured hardships for my
name, and have not grown weary."
(Revelation 2:3)

"Holy, holy, holy is the Lord God Almighty, who was, and is,
and is to come."
(Revelation 4:8)

"You are worthy, our Lord and God, to receive glory and
honor and power, for you created all things, and by your will
they were created and have their being."
(Revelation 4:11)

"Anyone whose name was not found written in the book of
life was thrown into the lake of fire."
(Revelation 20:15)

"Look, I am coming soon! Blessed is the one who keeps the
words of the prophecy written in this scroll."
(Revelation 22:7)

"Look, I am coming soon! My reward is with me, and I will
give to each person according to what they have done."
(Revelation 22:12)

"He who testifies to these things says, 'Yes, I am coming soon.' Amen. Come, Lord Jesus. The grace of the Lord Jesus be with God's people. Amen."
(Revelation 22:20-21)

"THE LORD'S PRAYER"

"Our Father in heaven, hallowed be your name, your kingdom come, your will be done, on earth as it is in heaven. Give us today our daily bread. And forgive us our debts, as we also have forgiven our debtors. And lead us not into temptation, but deliver us from the evil one."
(Matthew 6:9-13)

"THE 23RD PSALM"

"The Lord is my shepherd, I lack nothing. He makes me lie down in green pastures, he leads me beside quiet waters, he refreshes my soul. He guides me along the right paths for his name's sake. Even though I walk through the darkest valley, I will fear no evil, for you are with me; your rod and your staff, they comfort me. You prepare a table before me in the presence of my enemies. You anoint my head with oil; my cup overflows. Surely your goodness and love will follow me all the days of my life, and I will dwell in the house of the Lord forever."
(Psalm 23:1-6)

"CARL'S HEALING PSALM"

"I waited patiently for the Lord; he turned to me and heard my cry. He lifted me out of the slimy pit, out of the mud and mire; he set my feet on a rock and gave me a firm place to stand. He put a new song in my mouth, a hymn of praise to our God. Many will see and fear the Lord and put their trust in him. Blessed is the one who trusts in the Lord, who does not look to the proud, to those who turn aside to false gods.

Many, Lord my God, are the wonders you have done, the things you planned for us. None can compare with you; were I to speak and tell of your deeds, they would be too many to declare. Sacrifice and offering you did not desire—but my ears you have opened—burnt offerings and sin offerings you did not require. Then I said, 'Here I am, I have come—it is written about me in the scroll. I desire to do your will, my God; your law is within my heart.' I proclaim your saving acts in the great assembly; I do not seal my lips, Lord, as you know. I do not hide your righteousness in my heart; I speak of your faithfulness and your saving help. I do not conceal your love and your faithfulness from the great assembly. Do not withhold your mercy from me, Lord; may your love and faithfulness always protect me. For troubles without number surround me; my sins have overtaken me, and I cannot see. They are more than the hairs of my head, and my heart fails within me. Be pleased to save me, Lord; come quickly, Lord, to help me. May all who want to take my life be put to shame and confusion; may all who desire my ruin be turned back in disgrace. May those who say to me, 'Aha! Aha!' be appalled at their own shame. But may all who seek you rejoice and be glad in you; may those who long for your saving help always say, 'The Lord is great!' But as for me, I am poor and needy; may the Lord think of me. You are my help and my deliverer; you are my God, do not delay."

(Psalm 40:1-17)

"A TIME FOR EVERYTHING"

"There is a time for everything, and a season for every activity under the heavens: a time to be born and a time to die, a time to plant and a time to uproot, a time to kill and a time to heal, a time to tear down and a time to build, a time to weep and a time to laugh, a time to mourn and a time to dance, a time to scatter stones and a time to gather them, a time to embrace and a time to refrain from embracing, a time to search and a time to give up, a time to keep and a time to throw away, a time to tear and a time to mend, a time to be silent and a time to speak, a time to love and a time to hate, a time for war and a time for peace."
(Ecclesiastes 3:1-8)

"THE BEATITUDES"

"Blessed are the poor in spirit, for theirs is the kingdom of heaven. Blessed are those who mourn, for they will be comforted. Blessed are the meek, for they will inherit the earth. Blessed are those who hunger and thirst for righteousness, for they will be filled. Blessed are the merciful, for they will be shown mercy. Blessed are the pure in heart, for they will see God. Blessed are the peacemakers, for they will be called children of God. Blessed are those who are persecuted because of righteousness, for theirs is the kingdom of heaven. Blessed are you when people insult you, persecute you and falsely say all kinds of evil against you because of me. Rejoice and be glad, because great is your reward in heaven, for in the same way they persecuted the prophets who were before you."
(Matthew 5:3-12)

"THE LOVE CHAPTER"
(MY MOTHER'S FAVORITE)

"If I speak in the tongues of men or of angels, but do not have love, I am only a resounding gong or a clanging cymbal. If I have the gift of prophecy and can fathom all mysteries and all knowledge, and if I have a faith that can move mountains, but do not have love, I am nothing. If I give all I possess to the poor and give over my body to hardship that I may boast, but do not have love, I gain nothing. Love is patient, love is kind. It does not envy, it does not boast, it is not proud. It does not dishonor others, it is not self-seeking, it is not easily angered, it keeps no record of wrongs. Love does not delight in evil but rejoices with the truth. It always protects, always trusts, always hopes, always perseveres. Love never fails. But where there are prophecies, they will cease; where there are tongues, they will be stilled; where there is knowledge, it will pass away. For we know in part and we prophesy in part, but when completeness comes, what is in part disappears. When I was a child, I talked like a child, I thought like a child, I reasoned like a child. When I became a man, I put the ways of childhood behind me. For now we see only a reflection as in a mirror; then we shall see face to face. Now I know in part;

then I shall know fully, even as I am fully known. And now these three remain: faith, hope and love. But the greatest of these is love." (1 Corinthians 13:1-13)

My mother, Arleen Lindelien, read me these scriptures for hours while I was in pain and suffering—they really helped me over the years. Our prayer is for you to use them to bring comfort when nothing else will work! Please take these scriptures with you to the hospital and to home visits! God bless you!

THANK YOU

"But thanks be to God! He gives us the victory through our Lord Jesus Christ."
(1 Corinthians 15:57 NIV)

First and most important, I want to thank God Almighty for the gift of healing and the miraculous healing in my body on Father's Day 2014.

I also would like to thank many people who, over my health journey, have used their gifts and talents to help me—in all kinds of different ways—to encourage and help me physically. A big thank you to all of you! May God truly bless each one of you and your families!

Physicians:

Dr. Kirk Morgan, M.D. Retina Specialist

Dr. Carmelo Panetta, M.D., Cardiologist

Dr. David Sutherland, M.D., Chief Surgeon for Transplantation

Dr. Raja Kandaswamy, M.D., Professor of Transplant Surgery and Vascular Access

Dr. Ty Dunn, M.D., General Surgery and Transplant Surgeon

Dr. Mohamed Hassan, M.D., Hepatology, Liver Transplantation, and General G.I.

Dr. Yvonne Datta, M.D., Hematology, Oncology, and Transplantation

Dr. JoAnne Young, M.D., Director, Transplantation and Infectious Diseases

Dr. Alexandra Kukla, M.D., Nephrology and Transplantation

Dr. Gregory B. Synder, M.D., D.A., B.R., Interventional Radiology

Dr. Gregory Beilman, M.D., Acute Care Surgeon, Transplant Surgeon, and G.I.

Dr. Assad Saeed, M.D., Assistant Professor and Endocrinologist

Dr. Olga Duran-Castro, M.D., Interventional Radiologist

Dr. Naip Tuna, M.D., Cardiologist

Dr. Satish Rao, M.D., Gastroenterologist at University of Iowa

Dr. Joseph Schuster, M.D., Podiatry

Dr. Sandra Montezuma, M.D., Ophthalmology

Dr. Brian Sick, M.D., Internist

Nurses:

Marci Siers, R.N., Pre-Transplant Coordinator

Katie Huseth, R.N., N.P.

Margaret Mork, R.N.

Beth Omen, R.N.

Becky Gunn, R.N.

Tony Sioco, R.N.

Paul Herinstein, R.N.

Shelly Kuzsler, R.N.

Brooke Noelle, R.N.

Darcel Lott, R.N.

Annie Dahl, R.N.

Katie Wenaas, R.N.

Kim Trulen, R.N.

Julie Breitbach, R.N.

Andrea Carrico, R.N.

Alison Heil, R.N.
Janet Boyle, R.N.
Carly Nelson, R.N.
Bridget Leier, R.N.
Annie Doyle, R.N.
Beth Hoffman, R.N.
Rita Schmitt, R.N.
Kate Remus, R.N. (who saved my life!)
Carmen Ellens and Kevin, front desk
Karen Norgard, R.N. (2004-2006)
Alison Valinski, R.N. (2006-2014)

CNA and NAR: (Nursing Assistants)
Krissy Viken
Tony
Patricia Kadrlik (our hero!)

PCA: (Personal Care Attendant)
Arleen Lindelien (2004-2010)
Shanna Fare Lindelien (2006-2012)
Rachel Lorenzen (2006-2014)
Collen Heikkila, R.N. (2006-2013)
Jo-Ann Dubbels, R.N. (2006-2013)

Social Workers:
Angie Howard
Jan Misuka

Transplant Team:
Cat Gese
Alan, Michelle, and Joan
Maureen, R.N., Post-Transplant Coordinator
Erin, R.N.

Hospital Receptionist:

Deb, Receptionist at the University of Minnesota Hospital

Fairview Home Infusion:

Lori, Pharmacist

Sandy, Pharmacist

My Family:

My brothers, Ted and Tom, thank you for your prayers and words of encouragement!

My sisters, Linda, Lynette, and Liz, thanks for the visits, cards, and prayers!

Our children and grandchildren, thank you for helping me laugh and see the good in every day of our lives spent together. I will never forget the fun we had each day!

Mr. Scott Naegeli, a lifelong friend who kept me company for days on end and many evenings. Thank you for helping me through the simplest and most difficult times!

Ministers:

Rev. Jerry and Kathy Strandquist, Cedar Valley Church, Bloomington, MN

Rev. Kenneth and Joyce Broadus (Brother and Sister B.), Cedar Lake Christian Assembly, Biloxi, MS

Rev. Alex and Judith Clattenburg, Church In The Son, Orlando, FL

Steven and Joy Strang, CEO and CFO at Charisma Media, Lake Mary, FL

Rev. Lowell and Connie Lundstrom, Celebration Church, Lakeville, MN

Rev. Clarence and Vicki St. John, Superintendent, Minnesota District Council of the A/G

Rev. Roger and Myrna Stacy, M.D.O., Minnesota Church Multiplication Network

Rev. Steve West, M.D.O., Hospital Chaplain

Rev. Kent and Becky Boyum, Christian Life Church, Farmington, MN

Our friends at Christian Life Church in Farmington—your weekly and daily prayers over the years for DeeDee and me have brought us through many high mountaintops and some dark valleys. We thank God for each of you, dear friends!

To the more than one thousand ministers in the Minnesota District of the Assemblies of God who prayed for us—whether it was once a year or daily for ten years—we thank you!

Rev. Jim and Julie Wideman, our dear friends in ministry for the past forty-plus years!

Thank you to all of our friends and loved ones across the United States and the world who prayed for us!

"The prayers of a righteous man is powerful and effective." (James 5:16 NIV)

I know that when we mention people by name, it is dangerous because we often forget people who are very important to us in our lives. If we have forgotten to mention you on these pages, please forgive me—it is not intentional. We thank you from the depths of our hearts for all of your health care, prayers, help, and encouragement. *We love you!*

ABOUT THE AUTHOR

Carl and DeeDee Lindeliens' life is a profound testament to the power of faith, resilience, and the unwavering faithfulness of an awesome God. For over forty years, the Lindeliens have dedicated themselves to serving in churches, pioneering innovative resources for Children's Ministry, and leading in Pastoral Care and Hospital Ministry. Their shared commitment has touched countless lives, reaching families of all ages, while always maintaining a steadfast willingness to advocate for those unable to speak for themselves.

Throughout Carl's significant health journey, the Lindeliens learned firsthand that adversity often brings with it profound opportunities for growth and service. Carl faithfully served as the Minnesota District Council's (MDC) Chaplain and Director of Pastoral Care for nine years until his passing. Now, DeeDee continues his legacy, serving full-time in the same role. She is deeply honored to offer care and support across 22 Metro Hospitals and Care Facilities within the Twin Cities area, as well as serving over 250 Churches within the Minnesota District Council of the Assemblies of God.

In addition to her pastoral duties, DeeDee serves as a Patient Advocate and is a member of the Patient Advisory Board of the University of Minnesota Medical Center. Together, Carl and DeeDee have two grown daughters and seven grandchildren, who continue to be a source of pride and joy in their lives.